GOOD BEING, GOOD LIVING

The Modern Model for Sustained Holistic Health

RYAN GLIDDEN

ISBN: 978-1-4834-2081-3 (sc)
ISBN: 978-1-4834-2080-6 (e)

Library of Congress Control Number: 2014919369

Lulu Publishing Services rev. date: 11/11/2014

DEDICATION

For professor Dahlin. It may have taken me ten years,
but I've finally completed your assignment.

To my beautiful girls. You teach me so much. I hope
in some ways your Dad can do the same for you.

ACKNOWLEDGEMENTS

Without my wife, Melissa, this book never would have happened. Her loving push set my feet on a path I had forgotten. Her support kept me walking during the times I wanted to give up. Her example inspired me to overcome hurdles, never make excuses, and always keep going. For this I am forever grateful.

Thank you to all of my teachers throughout the years. Whether it has been in your classrooms or in the words of your books or lectures, you have inspired and taught me so much. To April Anderson: without your skill as an editor and wisdom as a writer, the jumbled thoughts in my mind would not make much sense on a written page.

CONTENTS

INTRODUCTION

Do you have what it takes to be healthy?

"It's more important to know what kind of patient has a disease than what kind of disease a patient has."
— Hippocrates

Below is a modification of a blog I wrote a while back. When I first wrote the blog, I identified two key factors of "being healthy": mindfulness and discipline. After further reflection, I realized that I had left out a third factor that was quite literally staring me in the face on numerous occasions: education. Without educating ourselves, it is difficult to know what actions to take and/or how to direct those actions (discipline). I've changed *mindfulness* to *awareness* since it fits with my acronym, AED. For those of you who are in the fitness or medical field, you probably know AED as an Automated External Defibrillator. This devise sends an electrical charge to jumpstart the heart of a trauma patient without a pulse. It's seen as one of the most valuable tools to save a person's life if he or she doesn't have a heart beat and is not in a hospital or medical facility. For my use, AED saves your health, so in a preventative way, saves your life. So what is needed to be healthy? Awareness, Education, and Discipline. Let's explore!

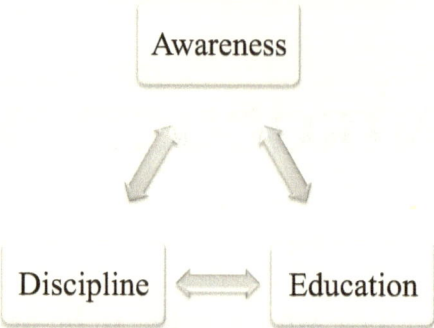

Should you cross-fit, cross train or weight train; run or swim; yoga or Pilates; reformer or mat; machines or aerobics; blades or bars; P-90X or TRX? Should you be a vegetarian or vegan, a pescetarian or paleo, gluten free or whole grains, Kombucha or Suja, coffee or tea? Salt is bad, but sea salt is good. Fish is good, but mercury is bad.

With so many choices and so many "right" answers, it becomes harder to answer the question of whether or not you have what it takes to be healthy. While the FDA pumps out food pyramids on what to eat, the CDC pumps out charts of a growing trend of obesity in America. It isn't hard to find facts and research to support the claim that people are getting bigger and bigger, and sicker and sicker. If we have so many solutions, what gives?

What seems to be apparent to me is the simple fact that in today's health and fitness world, robust health requires at the very minimum three very important things: awareness, education, and discipline.

We exist as a part of a universe so divinely complex, dynamic, and interconnected that an effect is almost never the direct result of a singular independent cause. Yet, when it comes to our health, it seems that we want to simplify human complexity in order for a particular modality to be "the cure." "Just do [insert product/modality here], and you will be the healthiest you've ever been." Ha! Why, then, is everyone so sick?

What does it take to be healthy? Life is dynamic; we are an expression of life, so we too are dynamic, an intricate symphony of systems all striving towards perfect harmony with one and other. Like an orchestra, if one instrument is out of tune, the entire ensemble is affected.

Whether you like it or not, you are affected by the seasons, stress, relationships, environments, resources, and more. In order to maintain balance, to build health, you have to become more acutely mindful of *you*, as you are now. While your calendar may say today is butt burn and spin class, when you check in with yourself, you realize you had a horrible night sleep and are experiencing high levels of mental stress because of a pending work deadline that you're way behind on. In this example, butt burn may not be the best choice. What you might really need is some light yogasana or some breathing exercises and a good night's sleep. Maybe you notice in the winter months, with shorter days and colder nights, you feel prone towards heavier foods, broths, and fats, while in the summer, you prefer fresh fruits, smoothies, and light salads. The point is you're always changing. Being aware of the changes and adjusting accordingly is key.

Sticking with the example above, it's summer time. You've noticed your energy and mood seem to improve on lighter fruit- and vegetable-based meals. But are all foods created equal? This is where education is important. There's research to suggest your blood type could effect your reaction to certain foods. What about your Metabolic Type? What is the difference between organic and conventionally grown foods? This is where you have to start seeking out credible sources of information and educate yourself on what you've become more aware of within your body.

The final step is sustained action. First, cultivate a deeper awareness of *you* through awareness and education, and then put it into action through discipline. This is where the change happens. One of my favorite yoga teachers, BKS Iyengar, said, "Knowledge without action and action without knowledge do little to help man."[1] You can tune in and brush up on all there is to know about health, but the simple fact is you are alive, and the only real change comes from the application of what you've learned. This is achieved through discipline. Discipline takes knowledge and turns it into wisdom. The system is cyclical. Through discipline, we gain new awareness, and so the cycle repeats again, progressing us forward one step at a time to more complete health.

Awareness, Education and Discipline are the real keys to health. There will always be new gimmicks, diets, and trends. It's a part of the world we live in. Learn what is best for you and when it is best through these three practices: awareness to how you are now, education about what you are doing or plan to do, and then implementing the discipline to test your education, thus gaining new awareness. Health is not something bestowed upon most of us; it's something that is earned. Unfortunately, the old adage applies here. You get what you put into your life. Too many people want a quick fix, and so they find themselves jumping from one thing to the next, frustrated every time that the results aren't what the images on the TV screen or magazine page told us they would be. I suggest stopping for a moment, paying attention, and then focusing your efforts where they will truly suite you best.

I wrote this book to serve as a guide to help you cultivate the three principles of health: *awareness, education,* and *discipline.* Throughout the book, I've included suggestions, exercises, and questions to help deepen awareness of the topics being covered. My hope is that there will be enough interest sparked to trigger motivation and/or inspiration, the fuels of discipline. The seven categories I present in the following pages are a synthesis of nearly a decade of my personal education and exploration of health. I hope that they help you along your journey towards more profound health and happiness.

How to Use this Book

Each of the seven major chapters is divided into three categories: *awareness, education,* and *discipline.* The *awareness* category is a series of questions at the beginning of each chapter. These questions are designed to stimulate reflection on how the upcoming chapter directly relates to you. I intentionally didn't include any point system to the questions. The intent is not to answer the questions, get a score, match it up to some ideal, and then if it's high enough, claim yourself the king/queen of healthy. No. The intent is to get you thinking about your habits, current states, and possible outcomes. You will notice, however, that answering "yes" to more questions than not could be weighing in your favor when it comes to leading a healthy lifestyle.

The *education* category is just that. It usually makes up the bulk of the chapter and is the synthesis of research and personal experience. The goal is to gain a deeper understanding of the way your body works, how it is affected by certain influences, and how those influences and your many body systems are always trying to create a state of harmony. The education in these chapters is certainly not inclusive of all points of study, but will give you a great foundation to continue to work and grow off of.

The third and final category is *discipline*. Like I stated above, knowledge without action and action without knowledge do little to help you. The discipline section is the practical application. Depending on the chapter, it may include a journaling activity, breathing exercise, checklist, or some other practice to get you going.

The three pieces together, *awareness*, *education*, and *discipline* are the cornerstones of holistic health. It's the closest thing to a magic bullet I can find. Hopefully this book can help you understand and experience that you have all the answers that are best for you and all the power needed to apply those answers to improve your health and wellbeing.

An Interview with a Farmer

Do you remember the kid's song "Old McDonald"? He had a farm. And on that farm, he had a bunch of animals. Well the earliest roots of this song are thought to have come from an opera called "The Kingdom of the Birds" in the 1700s. It wasn't until the early 1900s that some semblance of farmer McDonald emerged.[2] I've often wondered what it might be like to sit down with Old McDonald, the early 1900s farmer. How strange the world would seem to him. With the technology of today, so much work is done by machine rather than by human or animal; with the surplus of food in a developed modernized nation like the US, it would probably be overwhelming for him to walk the aisles of a grocery store. I've wondered, what might his answers be if I could ask him some questions about his life and what he thought of the world today?

I think it might go a little something like this:

Me: McDonald. You are in great shape. Do you have a gym membership, and, if so, how many days a week do you work out?

McDonald: A what? I work every day.

Me: Wow, that's ambitious. But what do you do to keep your body in such good shape?

McDonald: Ha, I move it. Listen. I'm up with the sun and out into the fields. The animals need to be fed, which isn't an easy task. I haul buckets of water to the troughs, I throw bales of hay from the barn, and I spread bags of seed for the chickens. Once that's done, I have breakfast with my family, and then it's back out to work. Recently, I put a new roof on the barn and placed miles of fence posts around the fields. Food is always in need of harvest, buildings are always in need of maintenance, and animals are always in need of tending. As the sun goes down, the work for the day is brought to a close, and I'm in for dinner. After that, I like to read or play a game of chess with my oldest boy. I'm in bed by 10pm and up again in the morning.

Me: Being a farmer, you must eat all organic foods, right?

McDonald: Are there any other kinds? I eat the eggs from my chickens and drink the milk from my cows. I eat the vegetables and fruits from my gardens and drink the water from the stream that runs through my farm. My wife and daughters cook some bread, which comes from the corn we grow. My neighbor provides us with meat from his pigs and foul, and, in turn, we provide his family with milk.

Me: That sounds amazing. Don't you ever take time off?

McDonald: Sure, Sunday is a day of rest and worship. Occasionally, there will be a fair in town or a gathering amongst a few families out here. The kids play games, and we take a day to rest and enjoy the bounties that God has provided us.

Me: It sounds like a hard life. Is it?

McDonald: Sure it can be hard at times, but nothing good comes easy. It's quite gratifying to see the fruits of your labor literally grow before your eyes. I have an opportunity to work with the earth, get my hands dirty, put in an honest days work, and provide for my family.

Me: Mr. McDonald, thank you. This conversation has been an eye opener.

The world we live in today finds us battling diseases like Type II diabetes at nearly epidemic rates. Obesity affects one in every three Americans (34.9%) and one in six children (17%), with this number predicted to increase. What is obesity? The World Health Organization classifies obesity using a BMI (Body Mass Index) score. This score is a ratio of your height to weight and is determined using the following formula: *Weight (in pounds) ÷ height (in inches) squared x 703*. For example, I am 6'2" tall or 72". 72" squared = 5,184. My weight is 180 pounds. Using the formula above: (180÷5,184) x 703 = a BMI score of 24.4. Based on your BMI score, the World Health Organization places you into a category ranging from underweight through class-three obesity. Obesity-related diseases have been shown to increase when a person's score falls over 25.[3] If these numbers on the obesity rates in America are accurate, which I believe they are, then they are astounding and scary, especially since they are more than double what they were thirty years ago. We are talking about 104 million of the estimated 307 million US citizens are obese. So what's the problem?

How does this translate into dollars? According the Center for Disease Control (CDC), healthcare costs related to obesity in 2008 totaled $148 billion dollars.[4] Many, including the World Health Organization, consider obesity to be a disease. It is a major contributor to heart disease, hypertension, diabetes, stroke, and some types of cancer. Not as easy to record, but just as detrimental, are the emotional and psychological effects obesity can play on one's self-confidence, self-esteem, and self-love. Stress is the cause of anxiety-driven diseases, which at the very least disrupt our moods, but in more severe cases lead to psychological disorders. We are at a point of living with the greatest technologies the world has ever seen. The invention of vaccinations enabled us to nearly eradicate diseases like polio, measles, rubella and more; however, our new way of living has only led to, in many ways, slower more painful deaths. If we judge life by its mere quantity, then we have improved, but what about the quality? I see more and more of what I call "the living dead"—people with the vitality sucked out of them from poor diet, lack of exercise, mental and emotional stress, and a complete absence of any Spirituality. They walk around in their body suits, but deep inside, they're growing more and more empty. Sure, their heart is beating, their lungs are breathing, but the life within them is all but gone.

So what's the solution? Well, it's a difficult question to answer, one I've found myself studying for nearly a decade now. By reflecting upon the blue-collar workers of the past, in particular the farmer, I found the answer that I share in this book. It seems the farmer or farmers have the solution, not just in their way of living, but also in their name.

Philosopher and author Mortimer Adler wrote a book entitled *A Guidebook to Learning*. In it, he writes about the arts and sciences. The arts he divides into two categories: fine arts and useful arts. The fine arts, he says, are all things that produce objects for our enjoyment. The useful arts are the things that can be utilized to accomplish whatever purpose they are desired to serve.[5] Within the useful arts, he specifically addresses the arts of farming, healing, and teaching:

> The other set of skills in the sphere of the useful arts consists of three arts that are distinguished from all other arts by virtue of the fact that they involve cooperation with nature to help it produce results that would come into existence anyway without human intervention. They are the arts of farming, healing and teaching. The products of these three arts—food, health and knowledge [in the broadest sense for the that term]—exist or come into existence without the aid of farmers, healers, and teacher.

> Farmers, cooperating with nature, help it to produce grains and fruits, and the animals as well as the vegetables we consume as food. Healers, or physicians, cooperating with nature, help the process whereby animal or human organisms preserve or regain health. Teachers, cooperating with nature, help the activity of learning that goes on in the minds of students in the natural process of acquiring knowledge and understanding.[6]

I use FARMERS as an acronym. It represents: Food, Air, Rest, Movement, Environment, Resources, and Stressors. By understanding these seven principles, we become the healer or physician for ourselves. We then serve as an example by which others have an opportunity to learn, so we become the teacher. Sticking with Adler's philosophy, You can use this book to build a modern model for sustained holistic health and incorporates the useful arts of farming [as a metaphor], healing, and teaching.

In each chapter I will address one of the seven keys. The first five will look at what I call the "Q" factor. These are the Quantity and Quality of each. With respect to the first key, food, I've added a third sub category, preparation. FARMERS teach us how to improve our diet, increase our energy, balance our hormones, improve our moods, lower our stress, and much more. As I mentioned above, figuring out what it takes to be healthy has been a passion of mine for nearly a decade. I have searched for and learned from some of the best people I could find in the areas of holistic health, whether it has been through direct trainings or research and reading. I've studied, tested, and applied numerous techniques, strategies, philosophies, and methodologies. What I've come to find is that it isn't as complicated as it might seem. Like McDonald tells us, it takes a little hard work, and at the end of the day, it's worth it.

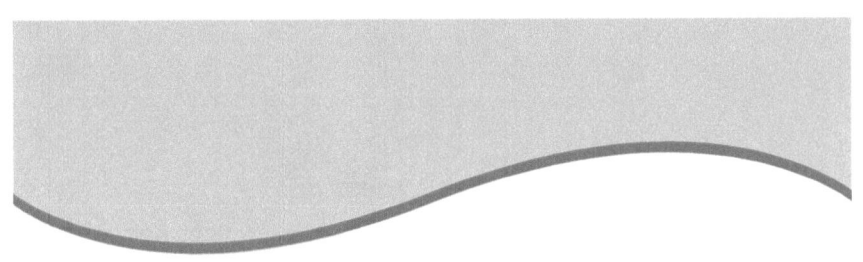

CHAPTER 1

FOOD: YOU ARE WHAT YOU EAT

"One immediately wonders if there is not something in the life-giving vitamins and minerals of the food that builds not only great physical structures within which their souls reside, but builds minds and hearts capable of a higher type of manhood in which the material values of life are made secondary to individual character."
– Weston A. Price, DDS

Awareness Questions

1. Do you drink half your body weight in pounds, in ounces of water each day? (example: 120lb. woman would drink 60oz of water a day)
2. Do you consume meat and/or eggs from sources that are free range, pasture raised, grass-fed, and hormone free?
3. Are you free of any regular digestive issues (gas, bloating, pain, belching, etc.)?
4. Do you avoid the consumption of foods containing white flour, white table salt, white sugar, or processed dairy?
5. Do you limit the consumption of drinks that contain caffeine or sugar?
6. Through the course of a week, do you consume four or fewer alcoholic beverages?
7. Do you avoid the consumption of food from fast-food restaurants?
8. Do you avoid the consumption of foods containing hydrogenated oils, margarine, or vegetable shortening?
9. Are you free of skin irritations or other allergic reactions from which the source is unknown?
10. Are you free of chronic diseases like type-1 diabetes, cholesterol, high blood pressure, and depression?

Education

Dr. Bryan Walsh produced a video series that I purchased a while back titled "Fat Is Not Your Fault."[7] One of the biggest points I took from that video series is this: you aren't what you eat. You are, however, as Dr. Walsh says, what you eat, digest, assimilate, and don't eliminate. I think this is a more accurate portrayal of nutrition and how it relates to its influence on the human body. Let's look a little closer at this statement and walk through it one step at a time.

You Are What You Eat

When it comes to food, the first of the front five keys to holistic health, we have to *mind our Ps and Qs*. This means it's important to look at three factors: preparation, quality, and quantity. Each one has its place in your diet, and each one is important when understanding a holistic approach to your nutrition.

Quantity

It has become more common in our society to only look at food quantity. When we do this, we're typically focusing on calories as well as grams of fat, protein, and carbohydrates. This is the basis of a calorie-counting diet. The idea is this: if you consume fewer calories than you burn during the day, you will lose weight. This is based off the understanding of something called your basal metabolic rate, which is a formula that uses a couple of factors, like age and activity level, to determine the average number of calories a person needs to carry out their necessary life functions for survival (breathing, brain function, heart rate, etc.). If you reduce your daily calorie intake of food (quantity) below this basal number, you will lose weight. It doesn't mean your heart will stop beating, but your body will start to eat up fat as a source of energy to keep things running. Specifically, a five-hundred-calorie deficit each day would equal a pound a week based on the assumption that a pound of fat contains 3,500 calories (500 x 7 days in a week = 3,500 calories). All else aside, this is a huge guesstimate and inaccurate in the first place. Many different factors make this generally accepted rule quite ridiculous if you plan to follow it as a method for losing weight. For more information on why you should avoid counting calories, read *Outsmarting the Female Fat Cell* by Debra Waterhouse.

A significant amount of research shows this type of dieting is extremely dangerous to one's health and in many ways quite unsuccessful as a long-term solution for weight loss or general health.[8] This is due to two reasons. First, it is unrealistic to think you will weigh, count, and point-rank your food at every meal for the rest of your life. Most people make it a few weeks, and the select few last anywhere between a few months to a year. There are just too many variables in one's life to accurately do this.

Second, this type of diet actually teaches your body how to more efficiently store fat. The body doesn't know why there has been a sudden shortage in food, and it is built to survive. So when the calories continue to go down, the body begins to adjust. Those carbohydrate sugars and proteins that used to be burned up or used for other things are now being converted to glycogen and fat and stored for later use in case the "famine" continues. This mechanism, without going into detail, has been built in over the course of human evolution. When the calorie counting stops, which it always does, and you go back to the same portions and foods you ate before the diet, your body will be more efficient at storing food as fat.

Fat Facts

Fat is probably the most misunderstood macronutrient needed by the body. The mass media has done a pretty good job over the past decade to convince the public that fat is *bad*, that we should eliminate it from our diets and our bodies. The simple fact is this could be quite dangerous. Fat is an essential macronutrient and is used for insulation stored in different areas of the body: under the skin (subcutaneous), on top of the kidneys, and in small amounts in the liver and muscles. Fat is needed for maintenance of cell walls, is essential for proper brain development in infancy and youth, and is used in the creation of essential hormones like cholesterol, DHA, testosterone, estrogen, and progesterone. Fat is also the greatest supplier of energy for our body through adulthood. For every gram of fat, there are nine calories. Compared to protein (four) and carbohydrates (four), fat has more than twice the amount of energy per gram. Fats are composed of building blocks called fatty acids, which consist of a chain of carbon atoms linked together like a snake, with an acid structure at the tail.

Not all fats are created equal. Some fats are required for health, while others are detrimental. Udo Erasmus, PhD, wrote an entire book on the subject entitled *Fats that heal, Fats that kill*. Whether a fat heals or kills depends on many different factors, including the following questions: What kind is it? Is it consumed in balance with other fats? Is it fresh? How has it been treated? Has it been exposed to light, oxygen, heat, hydrogen, acid, or metals?[9]

Fats fall into two main classifications: saturated and unsaturated. Unsaturated fats are then further classified as either polyunsaturated or monounsaturated. Sources of saturated fats are found in animal products, including milk, cheese, cream, beef, veal, lamb, pork, and ham, as well as some vegetable products, such as coconut oil, palm kernel oil, and vegetable shortenings. The liver uses saturated fats to produce cholesterol. Polyunsaturated fat is found in greatest abundance in corn, soybean, safflower, and sunflower oils, as well as certain fish oils. Monounsaturated fats are found in mostly vegetables and nut oils, like olive, peanut, and canola.[10]

As food is being digested, the gall bladder secretes bile salts that begin to break down the large fat molecules into smaller pieces called micelles. This process is known as emulsification. The pancreas then secretes Lipase enzymes that attack the surface of the micelles and break them down into the compounds of glycerol and fatty acids. At this point, they are small enough to be absorbed through the cell walls of the intestine. Once in the cell wall, the fatty acid and glycerol are rebuilt using a protein coating called chylomicrons to create triglycerides. They are moved to the lymphatic system and eventually meet with the veins, being released into the bloodstream. Because the fat molecules are too large to begin with, they need to be broken down first to pass through the cell wall and then be rebuilt. Once rebuilt, they are still too large to enter the smaller capillaries into the bloodstream, so they are transported to the bloodstream using the lymphatic system.

Within about eight minutes of entering the blood stream, lipoprotein lipases (found in heart tissue, muscle tissue, and blood vessels) are triggered by insulin, produced in the pancreas, to release and break down the triglycerides back to glycerol and fatty acids. The pancreas's release of insulin tells the cells to absorb glucose, fatty acids, and amino acids and to start building glycogen (sugar stored by the liver for energy), proteins (from amino acids), and fats (triglycerides). At this point, the fats are absorbed by the cells and stored as fat droplets. It is interesting to note that after puberty, the body does not create any new fat cells; they only get bigger. In extreme cases of weight gain, however, this may not be true.

The body is constantly in need of energy, even when you're sleeping. This energy comes from the food we eat. The body's first go-to energy source is glucose (sugar), which is readily available in the blood stream. Simple carbohydrates, like a candy bar or white bread, are metabolized quickly, providing a quick burst of energy. However, that burst is short-lived and is followed by crash shortly thereafter. Complex carbohydrates, like whole grains, are metabolized slowly, so they provide a longer more steady flow of energy without the crash. If there is excess glucose (sugar), it is converted into glycogen and stored in the liver until needed. The process of turning glycogen back into glucose is called glycogenolysis. If more energy (glucose) is required due to an increase in body activity/exercise, then the body can begin to break down the fat stored in its cells to glycerol and fatty acids (lipolysis). These elements, glycerol and fatty acids, can be further broken down and used as energy directly, or they can travel to the liver to be changed to glucose (gluconeogenesis).[11]

One of the problems for many when it comes to weight loss is that our bodies are incredibly efficient at using energy. Let's use the analogy of a car and gas. One gallon of gas is roughly equal to 31,000 calories. If we could drink gasoline, our human engine would get approximately 300 miles to a gallon.[12] Compare this to the modern day SUV, which gets fifteen to twenty miles to a gallon, and you are the greatest, most eco-friendly machine ever created. It takes time, and sometimes professional help, to shift our body composition back to balance. There are many factors that contribute to a person's weight gain, loss, and maintenance. A few of these factors include the quantity and quality of stress, lifestyle, food sources, water intake, and exercise. Weight loss, especially for those who are considered obese, is most likely going to be a change in lifestyle, not just a diet. The traditional approach of counting calories can be dangerous to one's health. This strategy for dieting is oftentimes fleeting—once the diet ends, the weight comes right back. Using critical thinking when approaching your weight loss and management is an essential tool to your overall health.

The general guidelines for nutrition provided by the Weston A. Price Foundation come from the study of traditional cultures and their diets.[13] Researchers noticed that many of the cultures observed had few or none of the chronic weight-related diseases suffered by a modernized society. Summarized, these diets contain (or lack) the following:

- The diets of healthy primitive and non-industrialized peoples contain no refined or denatured foods such as refined sugar or corn syrup; white flour; canned foods; pasteurized, homogenized, skim or low-fat milk; refined or hydrogenated vegetable oils; protein powders; artificial vitamins; or toxic additives and colorings.
- All traditional cultures consume some sort of animal protein and fat from fish and other seafood, water and land fowl, land animals, eggs, milk and milk products, reptiles, and insects.
- Primitive diets contain at least four times the calcium and other minerals and ten times the fat-soluble vitamins from animal fats (vitamin A, vitamin D, and the Price Factor—now believed to be vitamin K_2) as the average American diet.
- In all traditional cultures, some animal products are eaten raw.

- Primitive and traditional diets have a high food-enzyme content from raw dairy products, raw meat and fish; raw honey; tropical fruits; cold-pressed oils; wine and unpasteurized beer; and naturally preserved, lacto-fermented vegetables, fruits, beverages, meats and condiments.

- Seeds, grains and nuts are soaked, sprouted, fermented or naturally leavened in order to neutralize naturally occurring antinutrients in these foods, such as phytic acid, enzyme inhibitors, tannins, and complex carbohydrates.

- Total fat content of traditional diets varies from 30% to 80% but only about 4% of calories come from polyunsaturated oils naturally occurring in grains, pulses, nuts, fish, animal fats, and vegetables. The balance of fat calories is in the form of saturated and monounsaturated fatty acids.

- Traditional diets contain nearly equal amounts of omega-6 and omega-3 essential fatty acids.

- All primitive diets contain some salt.

- Traditional cultures consume animal bones, usually in the form of gelatin-rich bone broths.

Traditional cultures make provisions for the health of future generations by providing special nutrient-rich foods for parents-to-be, before conception, during pregnancy and through lactation and growth.[14]

What we can learn from examining these cultures is instead of counting calories, start to bring awareness to your quantities as they relate to portions and ratios of the three macronutrients: proteins, carbohydrates, and fats. William Wolcott, author of *The Metabolic Typing Diet*, has pioneered a clinical approach from about one hundred years of research that began with a man by the name of Weston Price. The basic tenant of the work is that everyone is an expression of his or her own biochemical individuality. What does this mean? It means that a universal diet concept is a bad idea because people metabolize food differently. Instead of following the USDA food pyramid, you should start to pay attention to what you eat and how you feel. Once you do this, you start to adjust your intake of proteins, carbohydrates, and fats in any given meal. The manipulation of these three variables can have dramatic effects on your mood, feelings of satiety, energy, digestion, and more. Wolcott developed a test to determine an individual's "Metabolic Type" and then suggests a diet based off of the results. As a Metabolic Typing Advisor and one who follows the dietary principles of Wollcott and Price, I truly feel there is no better way to eat. Everyone is different, and each person needs to find the ratios, or portions, that work best for him or her.

Quality

Knowing the proper quantity is one-third the battle. Next you have to consider the quality of your food. What does this mean? How do you know if a food is of a high quality or not? I will tell you. First let's explore the word "food" and define it clearly. All high-quality food falls into one of nine categories: fruit, vegetable, nut, seed, poultry, eggs, dairy, meat, or fish. These categories can be more simply grouped together into plant foods and animal foods.

PLANT FOODS	ANIMAL FOODS *
Fruit	Red meat (cow, lamb, pig, deer, elk, buffalo, etc.)
Vegetables	Poultry (chicken, turkey, pheasant, quail, duck, etc.)
Nuts	Fish (ahi, tuna, salmon, halibut, snapper, etc.)
Seeds	Eggs
	Dairy (cheese, milk, yogurt, ghee, butter, etc.)

* For the sake of simplicity, I have only given examples of some of the more common meats and dairy consumed. This is of course not an exhaustive list

I will use these two categories when explaining how to determine the quality of your food. Plant foods of high quality are two things: fresh and organic. If you wanted to take it a step further and consider the environment, they would also be local.

Fresh plant foods contain more chi or prana. Another way to say this would be to say that they contain more life-force energy. If you want more life, eat foods with more life-force energy. If you want to be dead, eat dead foods. I will explain the difference. Picture for a moment you're walking through an orange orchard. You stop at one of the trees, and you see the perfect orange. It is firm, and you can tell when you squeeze it that it is full of juice. You pluck it from the tree and begin to peel away its rind. As you do, you can see the zest spray into the air, filling your nose with the aroma of fresh citrus. You hold up a slice and bite into it. The juice rushes over your tongue and even spill down your lips. Can you feel your mouth beginning to salivate? This is an important thing to note, which we will explore later.

Now compare this to the dried orange squares you find in the trail mix at the gas station stop you made on your last road trip when you were trying to pick the "healthier" option for a snack. It's easy to see that the orange off of the tree has more energy, more life, and more nutrients.

Consider the fact that a plant is a living thing. When harvested, it is removed from its source of life-giving nutrients, and so it begins to die. Think of an apple core that sits out on the counter. It quickly begins to brown and eventually shrivels. As it dies and decays, the life-energy within it leaves. High-quality foods are fresh. One exception could be frozen foods, as they can be high-quality as well if frozen right at the time of harvest and kept that way until consumed.

Lower-quality plant foods are canned, dried, and or highly processed. Processing fruits and vegetables can do a number of damaging things. Juicing exposes vitamins captured within the fiber of fruits to oxygen, which can destroy them. Slicing, cutting, coring, washing, heating, and more can also change vitamin content, enzymatic activity, and influence the body's ability to properly digest and assimilate the vital macronutrients.

High-quality plant foods are organic. In the modern farming industry, there are literally thousands of pesticides, herbicides, fungicides, fertilizers, and genetically modified organisms used either onto or manipulated into the foods we eat. Organic foods should contain none of these chemical additives, which have been shown in many cases to be highly carcinogenic, since they are designed to kill biological organisms. While chemical additives may be targeted to kill a weed, a fungus, or a rodent, you too are a biological organism, so you are not free of their health-deteriorating effects. Genetically modified ingredients are plants whose genes have been altered to produce desired results (larger size, resiliency to certain bugs or fungus, color variation, etc.). In addition, plants are altered to be resilient to toxic chemical weed killers such as Roundup. The seeds of these plants have been given the title of "Roundup Ready Seeds." Planting Roundup Ready Seeds allows farmers to spray their entire crop without having to worry about harming the plants they're trying to grow. This means the "food" has been covered in and thus absorbed these toxic chemicals, which you will eventually eat. It also means that more chemicals are introduced into the environment, including the water supply.

The science of genetically modifying organisms (plants) is still relatively young, so the long-term health effects are not presently known. However, there have been a number of studies showing correlations between the increased uses of genetically modified ingredients and increased reports of food allergies. While the companies responsible for the production of these genetically modified plants claimed that it would take over forty years for certain weeds and pests to adapt or become resilient to the same things as the GMO plants, farmers see these adaptations happening in as little as fourteen years. Super weeds and evolutionary adaptations to certain bugs are already occurring. On top of all this, many of the countries that have banned the use of genetically modified ingredients are yielding more harvest than the US. A high-quality food is one that is organic. Organic practices require more responsibility towards the environment. The guidelines are strict and expensive, so you know that any company or farm willing to put in the effort and capital to grow organically has a strong desire to produce a higher quality food based on more ethical practices.

Animal foods of high quality are organic, but in addition you should be mindful of three other things when purchasing them: wild-caught, free-range, or pasture-raised.

Wild-caught refers to either a land animal (deer, rabbit, duck, etc.) that has been hunted and caught in its natural environment or, in the case of fish, out in an open ocean or river. In terms of fish, wild-caught means they are not scooped out of an aquatic farm where they probably lived with hundreds, if not thousands, of other fish in a relatively small container. Additionally, some species of fish are now being genetically altered to produce larger sizes, to have higher or lower fat content, or to remove undesirable natural traits. Wild caught fish would not have any of alterations. One other aspect to consideration is the location of the catch. As we continue to pollute our oceans and waterways, not all wild-caught fish is necessarily "healthy." Swimming in toxic waters or sewage would not be a desired location for the fish or the hungry fisherman. I get our fish from a company called VitalChoice, whose product is cold-water fish caught out in the open ocean. They deliver their fish frozen in vacuum-sealed containers with overnight shipping. They also have a recycling program for their shipping containers, so they can be used over and over again.

Free-range is a term used with common game and foul (chicken and turkey most commonly). Conventional farming techniques in the modernized world has chickens stacked a couple stories high with one cage on top of the other. The birds are limited in their ability to move, spread their wings, and exist in their natural environment. They are fed a high-calorie vegetarian diet (not organic unless stated as such) and kept confined as such until slaughter, or, in the case of egg-laying hens, a majority of their life. The idea behind a free-range bird is that it is allowed to live out in an open environment the way nature intended. The birds can flap their wings, breath fresh air, and scratch at the earth. They can eat their natural diet plucking for small grubs and insects as well as consuming vegetables. Free-range poultry is not only more humane, but it also affects the proteins of the meat and, in egg-laying hens, the quality of the eggs, including the ratio of omega-6 and omega-9 fatty acids.

When considering the source of your meat, look for pasture-raised beef. Similar to the chickens, conventional farming practices can have cows in small enclosures, sometimes not even able to turn around. They too are fed a high-calorie grain or corn-based diet. There have also been reports of filler materials like saw dust and other animal bi-products added to their feed as well. This type of diet is actually quite indigestible for the cattle and can produce a condition of acidosis in the stomachs of the animals, who then need to be treated with antibiotics, so they can be kept alive long enough to go to slaughter.

In contrast, a pasture-raised cow is allowed to live and roam in open pastures, consuming a diet of grass (what cows are supposed to eat). Again the quality of life for the animal is dramatically improved because it is allowed to live much more closely to its natural environment. In bio-diverse farming practices, the cattle and chickens work together. The cattle essentially mow the grass of the fields as they graze. The chickens come in behind them and scratch and aerate the soil as they forage for small bugs and insects. The fecal matter left behind by both animals' serves as fertilizer for the ground, and either a new crop can be planted or the grass grows again. The animals are rotated throughout numerous pastures, allowing nature to feed them and providing a much higher quality source of meat, dairy, and eggs.

So what about Dairy? Dairy is a top allergen for many people, so if you are going to consumed dairy, it should be raw whenever possible. The process of homogenizing and pasteurizing dairy products turns a fresh food into a dead one. With the level of consumption of processed dairy in the US being so high, it is no surprise that it is one of the top three food allergens, along with peanuts and eggs (both irradiated). Cow's milk and goat's milk contain active, live enzymes that help the proteins in the milk be more digestible. The process of pasteurization is the process of super heating the milk to 154°F for fifteen seconds to kill any and all harmful bacteria. The problem with pasteurization is that it also kills all the beneficial bacteria and enzymatic activity. This is not secret information. There are a number of hospitals throughout the US that have banned microwaving a mother's breast milk before giving it to the baby because the heating alters the structure of the proteins and can render them indigestible by a baby.[15]

Homogenizing milk is the process of putting the liquid under extreme pressure and then passing it through a series of screens. This process changes the fat molecules within the milk to keep the "undesirable trait" of having the cream rise to the top of the jug. The larger fat molecules in the milk can be captured and reduced, thus producing 2%, 1%, fat free, or skim milk. This process can change the fat molecules in such a way that they are unrecognizable by the body, and so instead of being assimilated, they are attacked as a foreign substance. This is an autoimmune response that can create a number of different health issues, most commonly a dairy allergy.

Preparation

The third and final thing to consider in holistic nutrition is how the food is prepared. The process of masticating and heating, as well as methods of storage, can dramatically influence the properties of a food. Here are some general guidelines to follow. Make sure to use the proper oils at the proper temperatures. Heating oil past its "smoke point" turns it rancid, releasing free radicals. Free radicals have long been associated with certain cancers. The biggest misused oil is olive oil. Olive oil is low-heat oil, but people use it for everything. It is best added to steamed vegetables after they have been cooked or drizzled over a salad. Higher-heat oils, like grape seed oil, coconut oil, and palm oil, are better for pan frying and cooking.

Store your foods in the proper containers. Glass is best. Aluminum foil is the worst. Aluminum is a toxic metal to the body and has been associated with diseases such as Alzheimer's. Never cook or store foods in aluminum foil. When preparing food, it is best to use stainless steal, cast iron, or ceramic.[16] Teflon pans scratch easily, and those flecks of Teflon go into your food where you consume them. Heavy-metal toxicity is a condition in which the body has stored heavy metals in its tissues. These are highly toxic to the body and can create numerous pathologies of disease. Reduce your risk by avoiding the dangerous metals. Stick to stainless, glass, ceramic, or cast iron.

If you enjoy juice make your own fresh juice and consume it immediately after the fruit has been juiced. The vitamins in many fruits and vegetables oxidize easily, rendering them virtually unusable by the human body. This process can happen in as little as a few minutes. All these smoothie juices you see on the shelves at the health food store, might as well be labeled "sugar water."

An interesting point to make on preparation actually has nothing to do with how you prepare the food, but simply the fact of whether you are preparing it at all. Research shows that Americans are cooking less and buying more prepared meals every year. The amount of time spent preparing meals in American households has fallen by half since the mid-sixties.[17] In a presentation on his book *Cooked*, Michael Pollan references a man by the name of Harry Balzer, a food analyst and Vice President of the NPD Group. Pollan references Balzer as saying, "He [Blazer] thinks that cooking in another generation will be regarded as quaintly as quilt making is in ours."[18] Pollan goes on to explain that Balzer offered a solution to many of the nutrition-related diseases Americans are faced with today. Balzer told Pollan, "You want to know the one diet that would solve the problem? Eat anything you want, just cook it yourself!"

In summary when learning to eat a healthy holistic diet, always consider the following: eat fresh organic fruits, vegetables, nuts and seeds; eat wild caught, free-range, pasture-raised meats; and always *mind your Ps and Qs*. Looking at just the quantity of food is not enough; you must also consider the quality and preparation.

When my wife, one of our friends, and I started our business, MOSAIC, we did so to provide the environment and framework for people to develop their own uniqueness, intelligence, and power, so they can utilize their gifts in service to others and the community. We offer a multitude of trainings, classes, and coaching sessions led by certified professionals in the areas of health, leadership, yoga, and spiritual development.

Here are the MOSAIC ten keys to holistic nutrition I teach to the clients and students of our holistic nutrition program:

1. If your ancestors didn't eat it 1,000 years ago, you probably shouldn't either.
2. Eat non-GMO (Genetically Modified Organisms), whole, organic produce, free-range or pasture-raised meats, and wild caught fish whenever possible.
3. Store foods and water in glass containers. Avoid brass, tin, and aluminum, as they can release dangerous heavy metals into the tissues of the body.
4. Cook using stainless steal, cast iron, or ceramic. Avoid Teflon for the same reasons as number three above.
5. Consume appropriate oils at appropriate temperatures. Olive oil goes rancid at a very low temperature. Instead use coconut, grape seed, sunflower, palm, butter, or ghee for pan frying and high-heat cooking.

6. Avoid the consumption of soy. Soy phytoestrogens disrupt endocrine function and have the potential to cause infertility and to promote breast cancer in adult women. For an in-depth list on the dangers of soy consumption, visit http://www. westonaprice.org/soy-alert

7. Avoid consumption of sports drinks, soda, and energy drinks. Instead drink fresh organic juices, herbal teas, and clean water

8. Drink half your body weight in ounces of water each day (120lb. woman would drink 60oz. of water).

9. Avoid processed and/or fast foods whenever possible.

10. Limit or avoid eating the four white devils: sugar, salt, processed dairy, and flour. There are a multitude of health issues associated with the over-consumption of these four ingredients, including but not limited to obesity, type II Diabetes, high blood pressure, lactose intolerance, adrenal dysfunction, kidney-related diseases, and insomnia.

A note on water. Your whole body is comprised of about 75% water. Proper hydration helps regulate body temperature, eliminate cellular waste, protect and lubricate the joints, transport nutrients and oxygen to the cells, aid in digestion, help with metabolism, help organs absorb nutrients, and more. Some studies have shown that the loss of as little as 1% of water can compromise certain brain functions. To further display the importance of water for body function, let's take a look at where it is found within the body:

Brain = 90% water
Blood = 83% water
Bone = 22% water
Muscle = 75% water

Proper hydration is essential for your body to carry out its many necessary functions of nourishing and detoxifying its systems. In his book *Your Body's Many Cries for Water*, Batmanjalidge recommends, as do I, that you consume approximately half your body weight in ounces of water each day.

You are What You Digest

Remember back to when I asked you to imagine the orange on the orange tree? You may have noticed when reading that section that something important happened. You may have started salivating. When I lead workshops and trainings on holistic nutrition, I ask the students this question: where does digestion begin? Almost always the first answer is this: in the mouth. While this seems like the obvious answer, it is in fact the second place digestion occurs. Digestion begins in the mind. When the mind begins to think about eating, it kicks the body into the physiological gears necessary to do so. Once the mind has done this, then yes, the digestive process continues in the mouth. Saliva contains two key digestive enzymes: protease and amylase. Protease begins to break down proteins, and amylase begins to break down carbohydrates. While both enzymes are present, most of the work at this point is done on the carbohydrates. Amylase starts to break the complex carbohydrate molecule down into more simple sugar, or glucose. The process of chewing food aids in breaking it down, especially fiber, so that the nutrients can be abstracted. From the mouth, the chewed food travels to the stomach, where it meets one of the harshest conditions in the body. The stomach contains HCL, or hydrochloric acid. Here proteins continue to be broken down and the hard food turned into a chime or liquid state. This chime is then released from the stomach into the small intestine. The small intestine itself is actually quite large. If stretched out, it would be roughly the size of a regulation-size tennis court. It's referred to as the small intestine because its diameter is smaller than that of the large intestine/colon.[19]

You are What You Assimilate

It is in the small intestine, with the help of the gallbladder and pancreas, that proteins and fats are broken down into their smaller parts of amino acids and triglycerides. In an ideal situation, these building blocks for life are absorbed through the intestinal wall and carried throughout the blood stream to be used for numerous functions within the body. The small intestine and colon also contain some 100 trillion bacteria, ideally living in a symbiotic fashion. While billions of bacteria reside in the small intestine, a vast majority (trillions and trillions) live in the colon. These probiotics play an important role in fighting infectious disease; manufacturing vitamins, including multiple B vitamins, folic acid, and vitamin K; increasing the absorption of minerals such as copper, iron, magnesium, and manganese; increasing our resistance to food poisoning; playing a role in normalizing serum cholesterol and triglycerides; and much more.[20] What remains by the end of the journey through the small intestine is essentially waste material. This waste enters the colon, where any last bit of water is withdrawn and some last vitamins are synthesized. Finally the waste is removed through a bowl movement.

You are What You <u>Don't</u> Eliminate

If there is an issue with digestion and assimilation, waste material may remain within the colon for extended periods of time. If it remains long enough, it becomes toxic and starts to be partially reabsorbed. A healthy bowl movement should come out like a brown banana. It should slide out easily and not need to be coaxed.

Regular elimination of waste is an essential process to maintaining good health. A healthy elimination time or transit time, from mouth to bowel movement, is usually every eighteen to twenty-four hours. If you are unsure and would like to do a simple home test, eat three or four whole red beets. Note the time at consumption and note the time of red elimination. The beets will maintain their color, making it easy to see when they have been eliminated. It is not uncommon with the classic American diet to have a transit time that is over twenty-four hours. Two major causes for this delay in time to elimination are a lack of fiber in the diet and inadequate hydration. Cleaning up your diet to include more whole foods and hydrating with plenty of water can do wonders for your elimination and thus your health.

Discipline

Using the sheet below, begin to keep a diet log. Track the food you consume and how it makes you feel. There is also a space to record your ratios of proteins, carbohydrates, and fats, as well as liquids. Additionally, I've included an area to track your activity level.

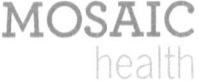

Water Intake: _____ Ounces

DATE: _____

Sleep Quality: GREAT   FAIR   POOR

MEAL	FOOD	REACTION (Energy/Appetite/Cravings/ Mental/Emotional)		ACTIVITY	DUR.
BREAKFAST % C: F: P:					
SNACK C: F: P:					
LUNCH C: F: P:					
SNACK C: F: P:					
DINNER C: F: P:					

DUR. = Duration
C = Carbs   F = Fat   P = Protein

Supplements:

Drink (other than water):

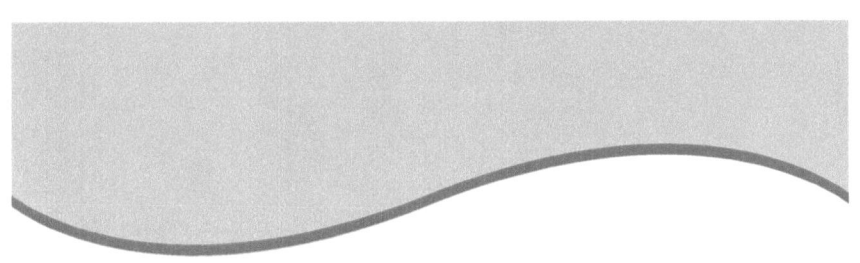

CHAPTER 2

AIR: THREE MINUTES TO LIVE

"The rhythm of the body, the melody of the mind, and the harmony of the soul create the symphony of life."
– BKS Iyengar

Awareness Questions

1. Do you pause during the day to check in with your posture and how it affects your breathing?
2. Do you use your breath to promote relaxation and creativity?
3. Do you have a regular breathing (pranayama) practice?
4. Do you recognize that stressful situations in your life can alter your breathing pattern and then create more stress?
5. When you take a deep breath, does it feel full and complete?
6. Do you know about how many breaths per minute you take?
7. Do you limit the use of air pollutants such as aerosol sprays, air fresheners, and chemically scented candles?
8. Can you consciously control the movement of your breath between your abdomen and chest?
9. When you breathe, do you notice a slight expansion of your belly as well as your chest?
10. Do you use the breath to promote focus and attention?

Education

Grab a stopwatch or take a look at the second hand on your watch. Now, take a deep breath in and hold it. See how long you last before you gasp for your next breath. If you made it a minute, you're better than most. Survival experts have something they call the rule of threes. Essentially what they say is that you can make it three weeks without food, three days without water, but only three minutes without oxygen. Our breath gives us life, and while there is plenty of science to support this, for years it has also been associated with the movement of subtle energies throughout the body. Athletes, martial artists, yogis, and warriors throughout time have accessed the power of the breath. While the physiological and psychological benefits to proper breathing have been a topic of much research, the average person only breathes with about 25% of their total capacity, taking between twelve to fifteen breaths per minute.

The Anatomy of Breath

Oxygenation of all the body tissues is paramount to good health. When levels of carbon dioxide in the blood are high, a message is sent to the brain to take a breath. The muscle fibers of the diaphragm contract, creating a natural massage to the upper abdominal organs (liver, stomach, pancreas, and transverse large intestine) as it presses them down and out to create room for the expanding lungs. Primary and secondary muscles support this movement by stabilizing the spine, opening the ribs, lifting the collarbones, and moving the abdomen. The internal area between the lungs, the ribcage, and the diaphragm is called the plural cavity. It's a vacuum seal around the lungs that keeps them from collapsing during exhale. Air moves through the nostrils, nasal cavity, mouth, and trachea. Upon entering the lungs, the air branches off in the brachial tree, moving into smaller and smaller bronchioles. The bronchioles open into the 300 million alveoli in the lungs. The alveoli pass oxygen through capillaries and into the bloodstream. Oxygen-rich blood moves through the body via the circulatory system, so it can be delivered to the cells and used in the metabolic process for the ***creation of energy***. The result of this process is waste, including new carbon dioxide, which is carried by the blood back to the lungs to be exhaled. Thanks to the pons and medulla located in the brain stem, this process breathing continues day in and day out without you ever even having to think about it. An interesting point about breathing is that it can operate either with conscious efforts or without. Try to consciously sit and change your body temperature or increase perspiration. You will find yourself struggling much more then consciously deciding to slow down and deepen your breath.

Quantity

As mentioned above, the average person only breaths about 25% of their total capacity at a rate of about twelve to fifteen breaths per minute. This number is referred to as the "minute ventilation."[21] Make's sense, right? The average male with each inhale will draw in approximately 500 mml Hg (milliliters mercury) of oxygen. 500x12= 6,000 mml Hg per minute. This, however, isn't really how much oxygen is actually received by the bloodstream. Anatomy of respiration takes into consideration what is referred to as the anatomic dead space. This is all the space from the nose or mouth, through the trachea and down through the bronchial tree until the air reaches the alveoli. This anatomic dead space is roughly 150 mml Hg for the example above. This takes us from 500mml Hg down to 350. 350x12=4,200. Okay, so the average male inhales on average 4,200 mml Hg of oxygen per minute.[22] In the body's endless genius to self regulate, this number stays relatively the same, regardless of slow, deep breathing or short, fast breathing. If you take slow, deep breaths, you will be taking in more oxygen per breath but fewer breaths per minute. The inverse would be true for fast breathing. You would take in less oxygen per breath but more breaths per minute. What this means is that for the average person living at roughly sea level, it isn't the lack of oxygen that is the issue, but more the breathing pattern in which the oxygen is received and how that breathing pattern affects other systems. The exceptions to this are the extremes of hyperventilation and hypoventilation. The former is a state of rapid, short breaths. If maintained, a decreased level of carbon dioxide in the body constricts blood vessels, creates muscle tension, and exaggerates sympathetic dominance. This is why the old technique of breathing into a paper bag when hyperventilating was used. It recycled the expressed carbon dioxide back into the body to help balance the system. This hyperventilating breathing pattern can be brought on by anxiety.

Why is proper breathing important, and what is proper breathing anyway? You began this life as one cell. As an adult, you are roughly 100 trillion cells, each one carrying out specific functions within the body. The cells create your tissues. These tissues make up your roughly 600 muscles; 60,000 miles of veins, arteries and blood vessels; and all of the nerves, sending signals throughout your body at up to 268 miles per hour. It is no wonder that we need to produce about 1.5 million new blood cells every second,[23] as these cells have a lot of work to do. If the cell is not properly cared for, then everything that follows in the system is compromised. One of the primary ingredients needed by a cell is oxygen. Without oxygen, cells die and subsequently all of the tissues they create die. It should be obvious at this point that breathing is important for the successful continuation of your life. Not only does it provide oxygen to the cells, but it also has a number of other physiological effects on the body. The massaging motion of breathing on the lymphatic system surrounding the intestines is massaged with breathing, stimulating immune function. This rhythmic pumping described earlier also aids digestion, assimilation, and elimination of food. The flushing of fresh, oxygen-rich blood through the liver, kidneys, spleen, and adrenals is essential for their proper functioning.

With a growing population of people experiencing stress-related disease, dysfunctional breathing patterns are becoming more and more common. Mental and emotional stress creates a sympathetic (fight or flight) activation in the body. One of the autonomic responses to this is to increase respiration. You might think that increased respiration would be a good thing. For the result the body is trying to create it is, but for long-term health, it is not. Picture it this way. Imagine for a moment you are on safari in the outback. The guide takes a wrong turn, and suddenly you're in the middle of a lion hunt. The crew flees, and you are on foot, running from a pack of hungry lions. Your body is built for survival. It is instantly going to set in motion a series of events, including, but not limited to, the following: increased heart rate, increased respiration, shunting of blood to the limbs, inhibited digestion, inhibited genitalia, dilation of the pupils, increased amount of circulating epinephrine in the blood, and more. All of these responses are designed to prepare the body for a relatively short burst of energy, whether it be for fighting the lions or running like hell to get away from them. The key term here is "short burst." Imagine you had to run from or fight the lions for a full day, days, weeks, months, or years. You couldn't. You would die. Though for most of us there aren't lions in our everyday living, the physiological responses to stress are still the same. What happens is the body, on a more subtle level of course, experiences this sympathetic response as a chronic activation to handle everyday stressors. While a certain level of stress is good for us and even necessary for our survival, too much stress over sustained periods of time results in both physical and psychological dis-ease. More will be covered on this topic in chapter seven.

A result of this prolonged stress is a dysfunctional breathing pattern. The breath becomes short and stays high in the chest. On inhale, the chest lifts and expands, and the belly draws in, as opposed to a functional breathing pattern where on inhale, the belly expands first, then the ribs and chest lift. This type of abnormal breathing creates a viscous cycle. Physically, the short breath stimulates the sympathetic response; organs and tissues receive inadequate amounts of oxygen, and the massaging effect on the lymphatic system is nullified. Dysfunctional breathing patterns also, over time, form postural imbalances. Some of the primary respiratory muscles are over active with others relatively inactive. These postural imbalances create inadequate joint motion of the spine and ribs, causing the joints to become restricted and stiff. Psychologically, a long-term sympathetic breathing pattern increases anxiety, perpetuating the pattern.

It is important to note that it isn't only stress that creates poor breathing patterns. Poor posture, physical trauma, and poor training techniques can also be a root cause of inverted or dysfunctional breathing. The key is to first begin to draw some awareness to the breath. Begin to notice your posture and your levels of stress throughout the day. If you exercise regularly, think about your breath in conjunction with your movement.

How much do you know about proper breathing as it relates to your training?

It is commonly accepted that there are three primary breathing patterns. Each creates a physiological and psychological response within the body. These three patterns are abdominal breathing, diaphragmatic breathing, and thoracic breathing. When breathing abdominally, inhalation draws the diaphragm down, causing the pressure to rise in the abdomen, causing the relaxed abdominal muscles to expand outward. There is little to no engagement of the abdominal muscles with this type of breathing pattern, as the movement of the diaphragm drives it. This is the common breathing pattern in babies, as they don't yet have the strength in other areas of the body to manipulate the breath. The result of an abdominal breathing pattern is excitation of the parasympathetic system, and thus it is a relatively relaxing and calming breath. This type of breathing also massages the visceral organs of the abdomen, helping to pump oxygenated blood through them.

With diaphragmatic breathing, the diaphragm draws down once again upon inhalation, but this time the abdominal wall is held taught and engaged. This engagement helps to stabilize the lumbar spine, and thus diaphragmatic breathing is the preferred breathing pattern for many movements, including those of yogasana. The result of this breathing pattern is excitation of the sympathetic nervous system with the mental effect being that of clarity and alertness.

The third and final pattern, the thoracic breath, resides primarily in the chest. The upper ribs and chest expand maximally while the diaphragms movement is minimal and the core musculature remains tight. This breathing pattern is the least desirable in most cases. It leads to excitation of the sympathetic system, leaving the mental faculties in a state of arousal and anxiety.[24] Try the breathing exercises listed below to experience for yourself the positive effects.

Discipline

1. Abdominal Breathing:

- Lie down on your back with your hands on your abdomen (a bean bag, bag of rice, or other light weight also works well).
- Begin to draw awareness to the breath, observing its quality and quantity.
- Draw the attention of the mind down to the abdomen.
- Begin to control the breath by breathing deep into the abdomen, allowing it to expand pressing the weight up towards the sky on the inhale and lower it down to the earth with control on the exhale.

Benefits: creates a relaxation response by simulating a neurological sensor called the baroreceptor, located on the wall of the descending aorta. The activation stimulates the hypothalamus in the brain to lower heart rate and blood pressure.

2. Alternate Nostril Breathing:

- Find a comfortable seated position.
- Place your middle finger against your left nostril, closing it about 80%.

- Holding your thumb there, take an inhale through your right nostril. Keep the nostril closed and exhale.
- Switch the nostril by placing your right thumb on your right nostril, closing it 80%.
- Inhale through your left nostril. Keep the nostril closed then exhale.
- Continue breathing in this fashion for a couple of minutes.
- When ready to finish, release the hand down, allowing the breath to travel through both nostrils.
- Take an inhale and exhale with the nose open.

Benefits: Creates a balance in the mind and body. Through a process of nasal laterality, this breathing pattern balances activation of both the right and left hemispheres of the brain, helping to focus the mind.

Quality

While the body may adjust itself to balance the amount of oxygen taken into the blood stream, the quality of this air is something that must also be considered. Today's environment is filled with tens of thousands of air pollutants, from cigarette smoke, to car exhaust, to hair products, to commercial bi-products, and many more. The body must clean all of these chemicals out, since it has no use for them, and so the detoxifying organs of the lungs, liver, and kidneys are strained. While it is well-documented that something like habitual smoking could lead to lung cancer, it is less recognized that the off-gassing of your new carpets, the chemicals in your hair spray, or even the lovely fragrance spray plugged into your wall outlet, could be contributing to long-term health issues. Below is a list of household products that contaminate your air quality:

- Aerosol hair sprays
- Aerosol air fresheners
- Chemically-scented candles
- Chemically scented "air fresheners" for auto and/or home
- Cigarette/cigar smoke
- Dryer sheets
- Fabric cleaners
- Freshly painted rooms
- Furniture polish
- Herbicides and pesticides
- New carpet off-gassing

The best recommendation is to breath fresh air on a regular basis. If you live in the heart of a major metropolis, you will want to find a park, at least, or even better, take a trip to the country. Fresh air is produced by nature, plants, that is. They provide us with the oxygen we breathe, constantly replenishing the atmosphere with fresh, breathable air.

If this is not an option for you, plan a trip to your local nursery and pick out some houseplants. Plants detoxify the air. It's a good idea to have some in your home to work as a natural air filter. It also isn't a bad idea to invest in an air filter. Research has found that there are thirteen common houseplants that can neutralize most if not all-indoor air pollutants. In fact, these plants actually thrive on the very chemicals that make us sick.[25] Below is a list of these 13 plants.

Botanical Name	Common Name
AGLAONEMA treubii	Chinese Evergreen
CHLORPHYTUM comosum vittatum	Spider or Airplane plants
DRACAENA fragens	Cornplant
FICUS benjamina	Weeping Fig
HEDERA helix	English Ivy
NEPHROLEPIS ex. Bostoniensis	Boston Fern
ORCHIDACEAE	Orchid
PHILODENDRONS, especially oxycardium	Heart-leaf
PHOENIX roebelenii	Dwarf/Pigmy Date Palm
SYNGONIUM podophyllum	Arrowhead plant
SANSEVIERIA	Mother In Law Tongue
SCINDAPSUS aureus	Devil's Ivy, including Silver Pothos, Pothos Gold and Pothos Marble Queen
SPATHIPHYLLUM clevelandii	Peace-lilly, White Flag

Another factor that impacts the quality of our air is environment. Depending on where you live, the climate could change dramatically from dry and hot, to cold and humid. These varying conditions could lead to dust or mold issues. If you have seasonal allergies, filtering the air in your house can also help prevent symptoms while home.

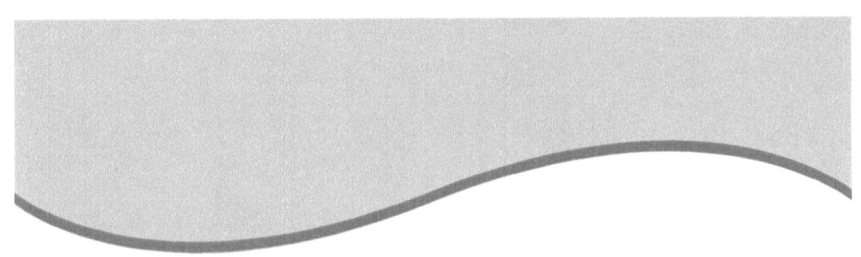

CHAPTER 3

REST: HOW TO EFFECTIVELY CHARGE YOUR BATTERY

"Every person needs to take one day away. A day in which one consciously separates the past from the future. Jobs, family, employers, and friends can exist one day without any one of us, *and if our egos permit us to confess, they could exist eternally in our absence. Each person deserves a day away in which no problems are confronted, no solutions searched for. Each of us needs to withdraw from the cares which will not withdraw from us."*

– Maya Angelou

Awareness Questions

1. Do you get a complete comfortable nights rest (in bed 10-11pm sleep well until 6am)?
2. Do you know the three different categories of rest?
3. Do you keep your television out of your bedroom?
4. Do you turn down or off most lights by 9pm?
5. Do you avoid all non-natural fragrances or body lotions before going to sleep?
6. Do you have a regular meditation practice?
7. Do you create time in your day or week for restorative practices (yoga, reading, relaxing music, etc.)?
8. Are you aware of how your last meal of the night affects your sleep?
9. Are you comfortable spending time in silence, without the distraction of TV, books, conversation, or eating?
10. Do you know how many hours of sleep you need at night to operate at your best?

Education

Without proper rest, the body breaks down. Athletes and trainers alike recognize that proper rest is an essential component to any effective training plan. Without rest, your body is deprived of necessary mental and physical repair. A common misconception is that rest is only achieved through sleep. While this isn't entirely incorrect, sleep is an essential component to rest; you will see, there are additional categories of rest that are oftentimes overlooked, yet still important.

We can divide rest into three categories: passive, active, and total. Passive rest is identified as a waking state using influences that help calm and focus the mind while resting the body. Active rest is similar to passive rest in that both occur during a waking state; however, this form of rest actively moves the body and mind. Total rest is quite simply sleep.

Type of Rest	Examples of Activities
Passive	Meditation, select reading and music
Active	Restorative yoga practices, light resistance training, walking, tai chi, qi-ong
Total	Sleep

Quantity

Total Rest

This type of rest is comprised of a single activity—sleep. The quantity of sleep we receive is regulated by two systems: homeostasis and circadian rhythm.

Homeostasis takes place all over the body, from body temperature, to acid alkaline balance, to blood pressure. The amount of sleep we need is also under homeostatic control. Think of it like a bank account. Every day when we wake up in the morning, we begin to debit from our account of available waking hours. The longer we're awake, the larger the debt. If we debit our waking account too much, then motor control, critical thinking, and verbal skills are compromised. One study showed that people who were awake for nineteen hours scored substantially worse on performance and alertness tests than those who were legally intoxicated.[26] Moreover, if we continue to debit this sleep account, we will need to make up for it with either a longer period of sleep or multiple days of more sleep.

Possible Physiological imbalance(s) caused by lack of sleep	Effect	Result
Reduced growth hormone	Plays role in puberty and regulating fat/muscle ratios.	Weight gain, muscle loss
Lowered levels of Leptin	Regulates carbohydrate metabolism	Weight gain, carbohydrate cravings
Impaired sugar metabolism	Regulates sugar circulation in bloodstream	Type II diabetes
Lower Cytokine chemicals	Used to help our immune system fight infections	Sickness
High blood pressure	Cardiovascular disease	Heart attack

The second system is our circadian rhythms. Circadian rhythms refer to cyclical changes in our physiology that occur over a twenty-four-hour period. Common changes associated with sleep are hormone levels and body temperature. Our sleep rhythm is regulated by what you've probably heard referred to as your "internal clock." Of course there is no hour, minute, and second hand spinning around in our head. Our internal clock is a group of neurons located in the hypothalamus of our brains called the suprachiasmatic nucleus or SCN. These neurons respond to external stimuli. When it comes to sleep, one of the biggest influencers of our circadian rhythm is exposure to light.[27]

When light hits our eyes or skin, it triggers the adrenal glands to increase the production of cortisol in the body. Cortisol is a waking hormone, which, among other things, increases heart rate, raises body temperature, and mobilizes glycogen from the liver to be used as energy. Cortisol levels continue to rise throughout the day, peaking sometime around mid-afternoon. Ideally, as the light of day begins to fade, so does the level of cortisol. In its place is a rise in melatonin levels. Melatonin is produced by the pineal gland located in the brain. The production of melatonin by the pineal gland is regulated by lack of light. Melatonin has an opposite effect on the body and is seen as a sleeping hormone. In a normal sleep-wake cycle, a person would experience a peak in melatonin between 10pm and 11pm. This would be an ideal time to go to bed. When our internal clock is set correctly, we experience a circadian rhythm of roughly sixteen hours of daytime wakefulness and eight hours of nocturnal sleep. This is seen by many to be ideal.

These two systems (homeostasis and circadian rhythm) work in a push-pull fashion. From the moment we wake, we begin to accumulate a need for sleep. The homeostatic system makes us sleepy, regardless of whether it is night or day. The circadian system, however, will keep us awake based on environment and exposure to light, regardless of the hours debited from our sleep account.

In nature, we would sleep about 4,300 hours out of a possible 8,760. This is roughly half of our lives. Eighty years ago, this number was down to 3,400; today, however, it is closer to 2,500.[28] For approximately seventy years now, humankind has been exposed to an environment changed by one of the most profound inventions of all time—the light bulb. With our ability to harness electricity in ways that power lights, televisions, computers, tablets, and cell phones, we have altered the way the biochemical rhythms of the body have operated for millenniums prior. We have evolved through time with a system that relies on the sun for energy. Because of this, it is generally believed that sleep quality is best when your sleep schedule is synchronized to the internal circadian rhythms and that of the external light-dark cycle. What this means is that you regularly rise with the sun, start to dim lights with the setting sun, and go to bed between 10pm and 11pm each night, regardless of vacation or weekends schedules. This harmonizes the two systems and allows them to work together, for your benefit, instead of against each other, to your detriment.

The quantity of rest required for the second and third categories, active and passive, varies depending on a number of factors, including environmental and physical stressors present at any given time. Because of the multiple influential factors, it would be difficult for me to draw a guideline around these categories. Instead, I would refer you back to the AED model of awareness, education, and discipline to constantly adjust and implement necessary rest strategies in your life.

Quality

Active Rest

Our bodies are built to move. Movement helps the body detoxify, remain limber, and improve joint health. Some types of movement drive the sympathetic nervous system (more on this in chapter seven), while others drive the parasympathetic system. Activities like restorative or yin yoga, tai chi or taking a walk, help to move the body in a restful way. A walk, depending on where you live, can also connect you with nature, allowing you time to breath fresh air and connect with the circadian rhythm of your environment. Making time for these types of practices are as important, if not more important, for our mental wellbeing than for our physical health.

Passive Rest

While the body is built to move, there are times when it needs to be still in order to recover. Passive rest consists of activities that may engage the mind while resting the physical body. Today we know that the brain operates at different frequencies depending on, among other factors, our activity or rest. Measuring EEG (Electroencephalogram) patterns, scientists can measure the electric current created by the firing of large groups of neurons in different sections of the brain. There are five major brain wave frequencies identified. Below is a chart outlining the five categories, frequencies, and mental states.

Brain wave frequencies from high to low[29]

Name	Frequency, Hertz	Mental State
Gamma	40-90	Memory consolidation; meditation
Beta	15-40	Normal wakefulness; strong mental engagement
Alpha	8-13	Non arousal; meditative
Theta	4-7	Dreaming; creativity while awake
Delta	1.5-4	Dreamless sleep

We can see from the chart above that the brain is the least active or most rested in a state of dreamless sleep (1.5-4 Hz). Theta frequency, the next lowest, is associated with dreaming and creativity while awake. This frequency can be found while reading or daydreaming. Above that is a state of non-arousal and meditation. These activities, reading, meditation, even painting or drawing, can be categorized as passive rest. While the brain is not in a state of complete sleep, it is not at the Beta frequency associated with strong mental engagement. Interestingly, it has been recorded that in deep meditative states, the brain seems to enter into a Gamma or super active state. This frequency has been associated with mystical experiences.

Total

There is still much to be understood about why we sleep and how much we need. There seems to be a number of different camps. Some believe more sleep is needed, while others think less is fine. One of the areas of discussion is not the quantity, but the quality of sleep. Sleep is categorized as two different phases: REM (rapid eye movement) and NREM (non-rapid eye movement). The latter is then subdivided into four stages.

Stage one is the state of drowsiness as brain waves begin to slow into Theta and muscle tension begins to release. Stage two is light sleep. In this stage, body temperature and heart rate lower. There can be moments of calm followed by bursts of activity caused by sleep spindles. The brain wave frequency goes up to more of an Alpha wave. Stage three and four finds the body in a deep, often dreamless sleep. This stage is sometimes referred to as slow wave sleep. Brain wave frequency drops even lower into Delta waves, and body temperature, blood pressure, and heart rate decrease even more.

REM sleep is much more active. The brain waves are fast and desynchronized. Heart rate and blood pressure may increase, and the eyes move rapidly in multiple directions. This is the state in which most dreaming occurs.

While there doesn't seem to be a unanimous consent on one's sleep quality, there are some physiological concepts that are worth considering. You can then use the AED model to take the new education, apply it through discipline, and gain new awareness to what works best for you. In sleep science, the quality of one's sleep is measured by something called the *sleep architecture;* this is the mix of the different stages described above, in different quantities, during any given sleep period. In the average adult, a normal sleep cycle consists of the alternating between REM and NREM sleep every ninety to 110 minutes, four to six times per night. It is believed by many that the average adult needs about seven to nine hours of sleep each night, with the ideal time for rest being between 10pm and 6am. This cycle is related to the body's hormone activity and repair systems that occur during those hours, especially the hours between 12am and 6am, as growth hormone and metabolic activity of the digestive system are at their max during this time.

Other research supports the idea that as long as a person makes it through two ninety-minute cycles (three hours) of undisturbed sleep, they will wake feeling rested.[30]

Discipline

How to establishing healthy sleep rhythms:

1. Wake with the sun (or approximately 6am).
2. Start to wind down, dim lights, turn off TVs, computers, and other electronics by 9:30pm.
3. In bed asleep between 10pm to 11pm.
4. Eat at the same time each day.
5. Remove major stressors.
6. Adequately hydrate your body.

7. No alcohol or stimulants (coffee, energy drinks etc.).

8. Keep a window cracked or a fan on to move fresh air through the room when possible.

9. Shower/bath before bed.

10. Aviod applying creams, fragrances, or other chemicals to the body.

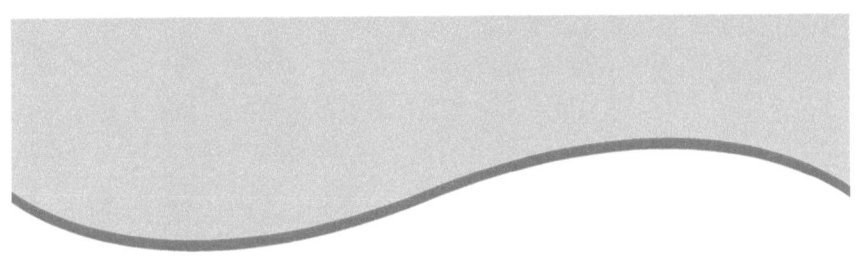

CHAPTER 4

MOVEMENT: USE IT OR LOSE IT

"Exercise to stimulate not to annihilate. The world wasn't built in a day and neither were we. Set small goals and build up to them."
– Lee Haney

Awareness Questions

1. Do you exercise (elevate your heart rate) for at least thirty minutes a day, three times a week?
2. Do you spend extended periods of time moving during the day?
3. Are you free from any chronic muscle or joint pain?
4. Do you feel strong and comfortable in your body?
5. Do you have the physical energy and mental drive to accomplish your goals?
6. Do you balance your workouts with both anaerobic (resistance) and aerobic (cardio) activity?
7. Do you lengthen your muscles, tendons, and joints via a regular yoga practice or stretching routing?
8. Do you experience a comfortable range of motion in ankles, knees, hips, shoulders, and neck?
9. Do you spend less than five hours watching TV a week?

Education

With over 300 joints and 600 muscles in the human body, we are built to move. Proper movement improves joint health, increases metabolism, strengthens muscles, increases flexibility, increases energy, maximizes the use of nutrition, and balances hormones. Improper movement/training practices can be catabolic (tissue-destroying) and actually harm the body and its systems more than they help. Understanding your current level of fitness and making proper exercise decisions based on this knowledge is essential to individual program design. Learning how to properly move through the six functional movement patterns of push, pull, bend, squat, lunge, and twist are the backbone to the fifth element in the FARMERS model.

Quality

The type of movement best for an individual varies quite a bit from person to person. Factors like age, physical ability, disease, injury, and structural imbalances should all be taken into consideration when deciding what type of exercise and how much movement is best for you. Because of the multitude of variables listed immediately above, it is impossible to write an effective all-for-one exercise program. Instead I've created a scale ranging from a person in horrible shape and working through a number of health problems to an elite athlete. I've included some general rules for each category.

Level	Postural Balance	Functional Mov. Ability	General Activity Level	Weight
1	Poor	Poor	Little to none	Obese (BMI >30)
2	Average	Average	Moderate	Overweight
3	Good	Good	Moderate to active	Healthy Weight
4	Excellent	Excellent	High	Athlete

    Related to quantity

Using the chart above, we would work from the left to right in order of priority. Notice that body weight is the last priority. Many times, being overweight is a symptom of another or multiple other imbalances. It is more important to fix postural deviations, build functional movement patterns, and slowly increase activity levels to get the body moving in a balanced, strong, and healthy way. Of course if weight is an issue to the extent of highly limiting movement, then it will need to be addressed sooner. Using all of the nutritional principles presented earlier in this book would be a good start to help with this. Another consideration is that there could be zones that cross one and other. For example, you could have good postural balance, but sedentary activity levels. You would need to adjust training techniques accordingly. So how do you do this? Let's look at each category individually first, then we can put the mosaic together.

Postural balance

This is the correct alignment of your joints based on the length tension relationships between the muscles and bones. This balance equates to a structure that is vertically and horizontally parallel to the line of gravity and the horizon respectively.[31] In 1961 at the Olduvi Gorge in South Africa, anthropologists L.S.B Leakey and his wife, Mary, found a single bone that resembled a big toe from the foot of a modern human. Their discovery was evidence that walking upright became a human characteristic as far back as 1.75 million years ago. This evolutionary shift brought about great changes to the musculoskeletal system, as the majority of the body's weight had to be balanced over the sacrolumbar and sacroiliac joints (the joints at the base of the spine connecting the sacrum to the lower back and hips) as well as the whole of the pelvis.

The bipedal position (walking upright on two feet) proved advantageous, as it allowed for efficient travel, freeing of the hands, and further development of the brain. The bipedal walking human could cover long distances over extended periods of time. They could use their hands to create tools, forage for food, and defend against predators. The freeing of the hands also lead to further development of the brain. The head's new position further developed the visual, auditory, and vestibular systems. As Patrick Mummy, creator of the Symmetry System for postural balance says, "Man could simultaneously run, watch for danger, look for food, and carry an object while following a thought process that involved problem solving and decision making."[32]

If your body is out of postural balance, then all functional (dynamic) movement created from this base of support will be compromised. These imbalances can range from an acute injury to more chronic problems. If they are not addressed, they become cyclical in nature. Trainers and physical therapists use the term *cumulative injury cycle* to explain this phenomenon. Altered joint motion (arthrokinetic dysfunction), altered length tension relationships (altered reciprocal inhibition), and altered dominant muscle relationships (synergistic dominance), lead to altered neuromuscular control, eventually Resulting in tissue fatigue, and so the cycle begins again.[33] Muscle imbalances limit the body's full potential for force production, compromise the joints, and increase chance of injury. It was this understanding of muscle imbalances that led me to becoming a Symmetry Therapist. Symmetry uses a tool called a palpitation meter to measure degrees of imbalance, rank their weight in terms of importance, and assign specific exercises to teach the body how to create proper mechanical symmetry.

Another useful modality is a regular Hatha yoga practice. When performed correctly, a regular yoga practice is not only great for stretching tight muscles and strengthening loose ones, but it also does wonders for your mental, emotional, and spiritual wellbeing.

Yoga has a special place in my heart, so allow me to digress for a moment. Yoga is a 5,000-year-old discipline. It is similar to many martial arts disciplines with one major difference. While many martial arts disciplines teach a student to neutralize or defeat an external enemy, yoga teaches a student how to defeat the internal one. Yoga can be described as the art of uniting and harmonizing the physical, mental, and emotional centers of the human being. It is a practical discipline for the dynamic exposition of thought and life. From my experience practicing yoga for over a decade and instructing over 2,000 hours in yoga classes and trainings, yoga ranks as superior in its ability to heal, restore, and balance all aspects of a human being.

A third modality I suggest is working with a corrective exercise specialist. The National Academy of Sports Medicine (NASM) has a program dedicated to certifying trainers on specific techniques for giving a comprehensive postural assessment and then working with self-myofascial release, active stretching, and muscle activation to bring postural balance back to the body.

The practice of self-myofascial release, or foam rolling, uses devices of varying firmness to roll the fascial tissue of different areas of the body to find and apply pressure to adhesions. Holding pressure on a fascial knot for approximately sixty seconds helps reorganize the fascial tissue fibers thus releasing the knot. Various techniques have been created based on the principles of self-myofascial release. For example, soft rollers like those used in the Melt Method developed by Sue Hitzmann slowly roll the tissues of the body, releasing them gently and with less pain. More forceful techniques like Rolfing, created by the Rolf Institute of Structural Integration, can use rollers or even stainless steel devices to apply more intense and forceful pressure to fascial knots.

Fascial tissue is classified as a non-specialized connective tissue within the human body (specialized tissues include tendons, ligaments, and joint capsules). Fascia is a complex system of organized collagen and elastin fibers that surround, pack, and hold all the muscles, organs, and other tissues in place. It has sometimes been referred to as an internal skin. This tissue can develop knots in which the fibers bundle into adhesions of varying sizes. These adhesions disrupt nerve signals to skeletal muscles contributing to muscle imbalances.

If you are not interested in taking up a regular yoga practice or are unable to find a symmetry or corrective exercise specialist, simply stretching your body on a regular basis can do wonders. Tight muscles become stiff and can build up lactic acid, decrease synovial fluid, and become painful. Regular stretching can help to avoid this. By stretching your muscles, ligaments, and tendons, you encourage the production of synovial fluid (lubrication for your joints) as well as help maintain full range of motion. Additionally, moving your body and stretching your muscles increases your proprioceptive ability improving balance and coordination. The Discipline section below outlines a number of popular stretch techniques and guidelines for practicing them.

Discipline

Contract Release: Hold a slight contraction of the muscle being stretched for approximately eight seconds before releasing it and stretching deeper. This is also referred to as PNF or proprioceptive neuromuscular facilitation. It works with the golgi tendon organ located at the musculotendinous junction (the junction between a muscle and a tendon). The golgi tendon organ is responsible for monitoring the length tension relationship between the muscles and the tendon. It will send a signal to nervous system to relax a muscle further in order to protect damage to the tendon. Many view this technique as the greatest way to increase flexibility.

Passive Stretching: As the name implies, this form of stretching uses the outside force of gravity as it relates to body position to create the stretch. In an example of a seated toe touch, you would allow your upper torso to relax or surrender forward and down, letting the weight of gravity stretch your hamstrings.

Reciprocal Inhibition: This is a primitive spinal chord reflex. When an agonist muscle contracts, the antagonist muscle relaxes. In the example of the seated toe touch (forward fold), you would contract your quadriceps in order to lengthen your hamstrings. This neural feedback uses the agonist/antagonist relationship to deepen a stretch. When one muscle contracts to take a joint through its range of motion, the brain tells another muscle to release in order for the movement to happen.[34]

Guidelines for Proper Stretching:

- Breathe freely. Keep fresh oxygen traveling through your body; if you can't breathe freely, you should back off.
- Don't bounce. Bouncing creates micro tears in the muscle, leading to further trauma to the facial tissue.
- Hold for at least thirty to sixty seconds. Allow your muscles to relax into the stretch, obtaining optimal benefits.
- Top to bottom. Work from your head to your toes or the other way around. Try and move your joints through a variety of planes of movement, especially your spine.

Functional Movement Ability

This is the ability to perform the six functional movement patterns under your own body weight with proper form and without the need of extrinsic support. World-renowned health and wellness coach Paul Chek made popular the term "primal movement patterns" to describe these functional movement patterns. He hypothesized that "selective pressures of evolution must have resulted in a human anatomy that was specifically designed to meet the demands made by nature. If one could not twist, pull, lunge, bend, squat and push from the standing position or could not effectively ambulate (gait), then chances of survival would dwindle severely."[35] While I'm only covering six, he includes a seventh, gait (walking).

Using the chart at the beginning of the education section, if you are unable to squat and return to standing position without the support of a dowel rod or the hand of a trainer, you would be ranked as "poor" for that movement pattern. If you could squat under weight without compromising form, then that would be ranked as "excellent." If we test all seven of these movement patterns, then we can score according to their success. Proper completion of two or less patterns would be poor, three to four patterns correctly would be average, four to seven patterns correctly would be good, and all seven correctly with the ability to increase under load or more dynamic movements would be excellent.

How We Learn Movement

Our sense of movement begins in utero with the development of the vestibular system. These receptors in the inner ear are responsible for keeping us balanced in a field of gravity after birth, but even before that are communicating information on position within the womb. This is why babies like to be bounced and rocked; the movement replicates that which was felt by the vestibular system before birth. Additionally, proprioceptive and kinesthetic nerves in the bones, joints, muscles, fascia, and ligaments communicate information about touch pressure, rhythm, and vibration, teaching us about our environment through our movement.[36]

After birth we develop through a series of movement patterns. At first we effectively have six limbs: head, two arms, two legs, and a tail. Our movement occurs from what is called a navel radiation pattern. The navel is the center of axis from which movement radiates out. The nerves of the limbs have not yet myelinated (protective sheath around the nerve that amplifies and directs its signals to skeletal muscles), and so they flail around wildly. Occasionally, all four limbs will rapidly extend out, even startling the newborn. This is the navel radiation pattern in action.

By flexing and extending our head and tail, we begin to wiggle around on our backs and strengthen the muscles of the neck and spine. This flexion/extension movement of the head is further strengthened in the sucking pattern. A newborn will go to mothers breast almost immediately after birth to nurse. This instinctual movement is for nourishment, but it also engages the muscles of the spine, starting the process of building a foundation for later movement.

Once a baby can role over, the next instinct is to lift the head and begin a push pattern, evolving the child's inner awareness to weight, gravity, balance, and movement. Pressing away from the earth is a powerful movement of independence and autonomy for an individual. Following the push pattern is a reach-and-pull pattern. Here the child starts to develop a curiosity about the world. With the head lifting, along with the development of the ears and eyes, the reach and pull movements develop as a way to explore.[37]

From here the movements build upon one another until the child moves towards an upright position, which involves a *squat* position and finally a *gate*. Using the hands as a base for support against a fixed object, a child will *push* with the legs as a way to reach and *pull* with the arms. The vestibular system continues to develop and establish an understanding of the body in space against the force of gravity. Once steady on their feet, gate will begin. This requires a static postural balance to then be integrated into dynamic movement.

In order to maintain an upright position, the body needs to have developed both righting and equilibrium reflexes. The majority of righting reflexes are built into our nervous system by the age of three. Righting reflexes keep the head in a normal position and right the body to a normal position. They tend to be dominant when moving across a fixed or stable surface. In contrast, equilibrium reflexes do the same, but are more dominant when the surface below us moves.[38] Further developing these reflexes can be achieved through proper exercise selection.

You can see from a developmental standpoint that a majority of the primal or functional movement patterns are present from the very beginning of our lives. These patterns have been built in through hundreds of thousands, if not millions, of years and are important for humans to perform correctly in order to move efficiently.

General Activity Level

The Harris Benedict Formula is a formula used to determine one's Basal Metabolic Rate (BMR). This formula roughly shows how many calories a person burns during a day to maintain general life functions. The scale I created in the table above is roughly based off of the guidelines the Harris Benedict Formula uses to calculate levels of activity. It is of no concern to me how this relates to calorie burning. More important is that the body moves. The categories are as follows: little to no exercise, moderate: one to three days of exercise; moderate to active: three to five days of exercise; and high: six to seven days of exercise. We will consider exercise, active movement of the body, for thirty minutes or more. Ideally, this movement takes you through a series of functional movement patterns and/or elevates your heart rate above its normal BPM (beats per minute). Below is a list of possible activities you can start doing right now to get your body moving:

Walking	Jogging
Running	Riding a Bike
Swimming	Stairs
Tennis	Golf
Tai Chi	Yoga
Qi Gong	Basketball
Volley Ball	Surfing
Paddle Boarding	Hiking
Resistance Training	

Weight

"Healthy weight" is typically classified in training using something called a Body Mass Index (BMI). This is a number calculated on the ratio of a person's weight to their height. A person with a body mass index below twenty-five is considered a healthy weight with anything over thirty considered obese.

As mentioned above, weight is the last concern. If you can fix postural imbalances, correct functional movement patterns, slowly increase activity levels, and follow all of the previous keys to healthy nutrition, breathing, and rest, then your weight will balance itself out to what is best for you.

Quantity

The quantity of exercise should and will vary from person to person, depending on the current quality of the individual's posture, functional movement ability, current activity level, and weight. Program design is the science of creating exercise routines that use a number of categories to determine overall quantity, or, in training terms, volume of an exercise routine. Sets, reps, intensity, time, and tempo are all examples of the variables used to generate a routine. If you are serious about starting a training routine, it's best to work with a professional. However, if you don't have the resources (discussed later), then here are some general guidelines to get started:

1. Fix posture first. Use the assessment and exercises shown earlier to correct deviations.
2. Start slow and build up. Make sure you can perform the six functional movement patterns with proper form under your own body weight in accordance with the guidelines listed above.
3. Integrate some cardio: swim, walk, jog, run, cycle, recreational sport, etc., to increase your activity.
4. Train smarter not harder. Slow down and be mindful of your movements.
5. Train with a friend or significant other to get feedback, support, and accountability.
6. Be persistent.
7. Follow all the guidelines outlined in the previous *food, air,* and *rest* chapters.

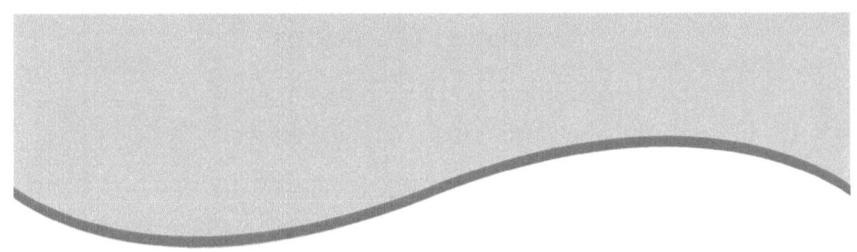

CHAPTER 5

ENVIRONMENT: YOU LIVE IN THREE WORLDS

"Rowing harder doesn't help if the boat is headed in the wrong direction."
– Kenichi Ohmaie

Awareness Questions

1. Do you feel your home is a safe place to live?
2. Does your home provide plenty of natural light and fresh air?
3. Do you have a quiet place in your home specifically dedicated to prayer, meditation, and/or personal introspection?
4. Do you see your home as a place to nurture yourself and relax?
5. Do the people who live with you support your health and growth as a person?
6. Are you aware of alternatives to your present job or work?
7. Does the work you do enhance the wellbeing of others and the planet without taking away from anyone?
8. Does your work require long hours seated at a desk or computer?
9. Do your co-workers support your health and growth as a person?
10. Does your job create peace in your life?
11. Does your job allow you to make contact with, or at least see, the outdoors (sunlight/fresh air)?
12. Do your recreational activities support or strengthen you physically, emotionally, or spiritually?
13. Do you engage in your community, such as attending a city council meeting or volunteering at a local charity?
14. Are you aware of the influences that different environments have on your thoughts?
15. Do you balance your recreational (fun) activities with your work activities?
16. Do you recycle at home and look to recycle outside the home when it is an option?
17. Do you choose modes of transportation that take the environment into consideration?
18. Do you use a reusable water bottle?

19. Do you buy your produce from local sources?
20. Do you consider the effects your work, home, and recreational activities have on the environment?

Education

Every day we operate in three different worlds: our private world, which is comprised of our home, our car, or any other private personal space; our professional world, which is the place or places where we do business; and our recreational world, which is where we go to have fun, decompress, or relax.

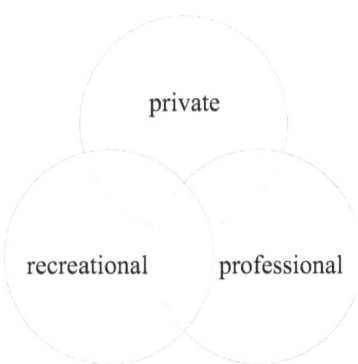

These three worlds make up our environment. They are not exclusively independent of one another, and oftentimes they overlap. As an owner of MOSAIC, we have a physical studio space. This would be considered a professional environment; however, as a yoga practitioner, this is a space for a recreational activity as well. Because there is no office space at the studio, I have one set up at home, so my personal environment also blends with my professional one. Each of these worlds can have varying levels of what I refer to as "toxicity." If one world or multiple worlds are highly toxic, then your ability to succeed in working with the first four keys (food, air, rest, and movement) will be compromised.

Private

The private world for most people is at home. There could be another private space in your life, like out in nature, but a majority of private time is spent at home. The home environment is a place where you store and prepare food, rest, and spend time with friends and family. Your home is ideally a place of reprieve. When in balance, your home is a place that rejuvenates, restores, shelters, and nourishes you. If your home does not feel safe or is full of toxins, then it becomes a space of stress and thus has the opposite effects.

Toxicity in the home affects both the physical body as it relates to the space as well as the mental/emotional body. Refer to the discipline section of this sub-category for a list of common physical toxins that should be recognized and removed from the home for better health. Physical toxins in the home may be easier to identify and eliminate than the mental/emotional ones. These toxins consist of unhealthy or dangerous relationships and unsafe or undesirable surroundings. There is no doubt that these toxins affect your health. Oftentimes recognizing and accepting these toxins requires a long hard look in the mirror and a real and honest understanding of what you're dealing with before a change can be made. If while reading this there is even the smallest part of you that thinks you may be dealing with these toxins, take some time to reflect. Seek out feedback and support from friends, family, or other groups. If you live in a building, neighborhood, or even a larger location that is dangerous and/or unhealthy for you (rainy, lack of sun, too cold, too hot, etc.), maybe now is the time to make a move.

I know first-hand that the home is rapidly becoming a place for more work. In fact, as I write this book, I sit at "my work desk," in my house, typing away. The key, as it is with everything else, seems to be balance.

The technology of today has allowed for greater flexibility in our work schedules. Work doesn't have to be done at a specific place or location anymore; it is more mobile and accessible than ever before. This flexibility could free up more time to play with our kids, run errands, or take a stay-cation.

However, the great benefit of technology is also its greatest evil. For the workaholics out there, there is no stopping. The boundaries between work time, recreation time, and family time have become quite blurred. People are texting at their dinner tables and staying up until all hours of the night finishing work projects. We've lost our ability to focus or even hold a conversation with another human being without thinking about or checking our phones and emails.

For those with a propensity towards lethargy, the following activities may be challenging: meeting deadlines, achieving goals, and accomplishing what needs to be done. The alarm going off at 6am doesn't have quite the same meaning when the office is downstairs and nobody cares about time, as opposed to driving across town when someone does care about time.

If you work from home, my advice to you is as follow. First, designate your workspace as such in a specific location in the house. Second, schedule your day the same way it might be scheduled if you were at an office and try to hold firm to the schedule. If you have small children at home like I do, you may need to revise the typical workday schedule.

The point here is that you have a plan for your day. There will be certain tasks that need to be completed daily, weekly, or monthly. Make sure time is allotted to them ahead of time. Third, put the least-favorite activities first and hold yourself accountable with deadlines.

Discipline

Use this list of things to consider when choosing or enhancing your private environment to ensure it is one that nurtures and restores.

- Location, location, location (climate, surroundings, setting, etc.).
- Find a space with exposure to natural light.
- Strongly consider the quality of the air you breath, both inside and outside your home.
- Find a location where you feel safe.
- Consider the quality of the water you drink. Depending on your location's municipal water supply, you may want to consider home filtration.
- Make your home a place to rest (maybe dedicate a specific area to rest and connect with your soul).
- Be realistic with your "required" amenities.
- Insure your home is in line with your values (size, energy consumption, location, etc.). More on values in chapter six.

Below is a list of common physical toxins in the home. Go through the list and identify the ones that are applicable to you. Over time begin to eliminate them from your home and your life.

- Aluminum: antiperspirants, cookware, aluminum foil

- Airborne chemical exposures: aerosols, air fresheners, fabric cleaners, herbicides, pesticides (see the chapter on air)
- Cleaning Agents: fabric softeners, nonbiodegradable dish washing soaps, nonbiodegradable washing detergents, all chemical cleaning products
- Hair/skin treatments: all commercial, nonnatural, un-organic, chemical products for skin and hair
- Dental: toothpaste made from synthetic chemicals and containing fluoride, chemical mouthwashes

Professional

Your professional world is where you go to earn a living. This is the environment of business, but may also be a place of recreation and, as in my case, a private/home space as well. The professional environment, when in balance, is a place that is productive, supportive, and enjoyable while also relating to your vocation or purpose in life. Toxins in this environment show up in unhealthy physical space: artificial light, poor air quality, and long hours of sitting. Mental toxins can show up as abusive superiors, mental lethargy, unrealistic expectations/goals, and poor team moral.

If you're someone who goes to an office or any location other than your home for work, the same physical toxins may be present as were identified in your private world. Of course careers/jobs vary considerably. For years I was a landscaper. I can't measure how much pipe glue and primer covered my hands installing irrigation or how many chemical herbicides I inhaled. An accountant would not be facing these same toxins, but instead might be sitting for long periods of time in one spot under artificial light late into the evening. Because of the number of variables involved with different work environments, the best thing to do is assess is the first four keys: food, air, rest, and movement. What do I mean by this?

Do you have access to good quality food? Do you have enough time to eat it? Is the environment flooded with toxic air (chemical air fresheners, fumes, stagnancy, mold, exhaust, etc.) or is it clean and fresh? Are there adequate breaks allotted for you to rest? Do you use them? Does your work require long hours and late nights? Are you stuck in the same spot for hours (standing or sitting)? Do you have the ability to get up and move around? Does your work provide any movement driven facilities or activities?

Discipline

All of the questions above are vital to understanding the health of your work environment. Below is a list of ideas to help you enhance your work environment.

Read through the list and check the ones that you need to work on. Once you've checked the boxes, assign a number to them in order of priority (one being highest priority, eight being lowest). Finally, write out a detailed plan as to how you're going to implement your highest priority into your work environment and life.

- Maintain self-care—nutrition, exercise, and relaxation.
- Limit or eliminate rescuing tendencies (doing for others what they should be doing for themselves).
- Directly ask for what you want and need.

- Exercise creativity and brainstorming techniques often.
- Accept your limitations with compassion.
- Recognize and understand the alternatives (there are other jobs).
- Be cautious to avoid defining yourself by your work.
- Align your work with your values.

Recreational

Your recreational world is where you go to exercise, relax, or spend time with friends. This environment is probably one of the easiest to introduce unhealthy toxins, primarily because of drugs and alcohol. It is not uncommon to have a recreational environment be a local restaurant or bar. While it may be a place to socialize and spend time with friends and co-workers, it can become quite toxic. When you're mindful of this, these environments can be a great place to let off some steam, connect with friends and co-workers, and have fun.

Other recreational environments often surround some type of sport: surfing, golfing, basketball, Frisbee golf, running, swimming, or biking. Others are a club, such as a book club, cooking club, or sewing group. Others include a gym, yoga, Pilates, or dance studio. The possibilities are endless. The point is that our recreational environments are places where we go to connect. We connect with others, we connect with the environment, and we connect with ourselves. Recreational environments are important to have in your life. Being in these environments can do wonders to clear your mind, exercise your body, and improve your mood.

Discipline

Below is a list of possible ways to enhance your recreational environment. As you read through the list, try to spend a few minutes journaling on each bullet point. You may find some new awareness around what recreational worlds are best for you and your health.

- Find things that fascinate you.
- Find activities that cause you to lose track of time.
- Engage in activities that make you feel free.
- Find activities that nurture you: writing, dancing, singing, silence, traveling, hiking, etc.
- Let yourself be light—be cautious of the effect competition can have on you.
- Explore activities that strengthen you physically, emotionally, and spiritually.
- Ask yourself this: are your activities in line with your values?

Connecting with Nature

Connecting with nature is a rejuvenating activity for the soul. We've all experienced a beautiful sunset, the silence in the middle of a mountain hike, and a vast star-lit night sky. Nature has a magical way of first showing us how small we are and then how connected we are to everything else. It is my firm belief that time spent in nature is essential to health and happiness. We have evolved over hundreds of thousands of years intimately connected to the earth. The brain developed mechanisms to wake us with the sun and put us to sleep when it was dark. Our survival depended on gathering and growing fruits and vegetables, as well as animals to hunt. Our metabolism built rhythms based on the seasons, storing fat in colder months when food was scarce. Trees provided the raw materials for shelter and ships. The nigh sky helped us navigate the open seas to discover new lands in which to live. In addition to being our container for life, the earth has selflessly served as a provider of food, water, shelter, and beauty. There is something very deep within us, hardwired to our soul, that draws us to her at times, sometimes lifting us up, and sometimes bringing us to our knees.

We have also seen the great power of nature—the force of a tsunami that can destroy an island city, the winds of a hurricane or tornado that can tear apart the strongest buildings, volcanoes that can burn and encapsulate anything in their path, earthquakes that can rip holes in the earths crust, and extreme temperatures that can destroy all forms of life. We have a responsibility as the dominant inhabitants of this planet to be mindful of the way we treat our home. Nature does not suffer from emotional dilemmas. It does not stop to consider women and children in the path of a hurricane. It will not warm the homes of good people while freezing the homes of others. The amounts of CO_2 emissions that enter the atmosphere are reaching astronomical levels, and with them the climate is changing. If we are not careful, our current course will disrupt the natural balance of the planet to such an extent that we will experience more of nature's great destructive power.

Consider your energy use, the materials, containers, cleaners, and even the food you purchase. Think about where they come from, how they are produced, and what affect that production might be having on the planet.

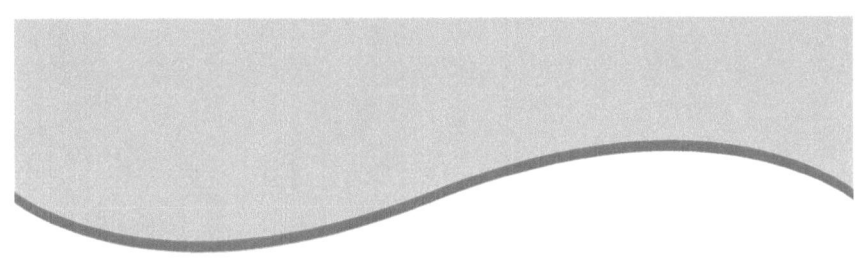

CHAPTER 6

RESOURCES: USE WHAT YOU HAVE; GET WHAT YOU NEED

"I have a low tolerance for people who complain about things but never do anything to change them. This led me to conclude that the single largest pool of untapped natural resources in this world is human good intentions that are never translated into actions."
– Cindy Gallop

Awareness Questions

1. Do you earn enough money to live comfortably?
2. Do you have a personal budget in place?
3. Do you usually feel like you have enough time to accomplish your tasks?
4. Do you keep track of events and appointments on a calendar or planner?
5. Do you have a network of friends or coworkers you feel comfortable going to in a time of need?
6. Do you have access to local and/or organic food?
7. Do you have the money and time available to join a yoga studio, gym, or other fitness-related recreational club or organization?
8. Do you have a particular skill set? If yes, can it be used to improve your health?
9. Do you have adequate access to food, water, and shelter?
10. Is your environment conducive to your health?

Education

My grandfather used to say, "Any job's easy if you've got the right tools." It's quite difficult to put a screw into a piece of wood without a screwdriver. Just like it's quite difficult to eat a healthy diet without access to whole organic foods. Some of the resources we need are all around us while others may be a little harder to find. In either case, in my experience working one-on-one with clients, there seems to be two primary categories of resources that feed almost all others.

Time

It's the one thing we never seem to have enough of. I've heard it a thousand times (no pun intended): "If I had more time, I'd go to the gym." "I don't have time to cook dinner or make my lunch the day before." "I would love to meditate, but I feel like I don't even have time to eat, let alone sit and breathe for a half hour." Maybe you've said some of these yourself. The thing is, most of us aren't actually lacking in quantity of time. We all have the exact same amount of time, twenty-four hours each day. That's a lot of time. What we're lacking is direction or discipline in what to do with it. It really comes down to a values question(s), not a time question. People have changed their entire lives to make time for new activities and eliminate others. You don't have to sell your house and live in a bungalow on the north shore of Kauai (although it does sound nice). Baby steps. First thing to do is get a clear grasp on the way you currently spend your time. Write out your day from the moment you wake-up to the time you go to bed. Include the times each individual event began and ended. Like any good experiment, one day may not be a good example of the larger truth. Use your journal and track multiple days throughout your week.

Once you have your data, take a more critical look at how you spend your time. The happiest people allocate the largest quantity of their time to the activities they find have the greatest quality. The final step of this exercise should start to bring up some questions for you. These questions are based upon what you value. If you're giving adequate time to the things you value most, usually there isn't a problem. It's when you aren't giving adequate time to the things you value most that the issues arise. The bigger, more important question to ask here is this: what do you value personally, professionally, and in relationships? Here are some great questions to help you get started.

Discipline

Personal Values:

- What are my physical health needs?
- What do I need in my life to be mentally stimulated and engaged?
- What do I need in my life to be emotionally happy?
- How do I want people to know me?
- How do I want to "be" in this world?
- What qualities do I wish to embody so that I live a life that is an inspiration and a model for others?

Relationship Values:

- How openly and honestly do I communicate with others?
- How do I prefer others communicate to with me?
- What do I offer the people in my relationships, to help them to grow as individuals?

- What do I need from my relationships to feel emotionally fulfilled? What do I offer them to feel the same?
- What do I need from my relationships to feel mentally fulfilled? What do I offer them to feel the same?
- What do I need from my relationships to feel physically/sexually fulfilled? What do I offer them to feel the same?
- How do my values fit with my expectations of others in my relationships?
- What kind of responsibility do I want in a relationship with my friends, co-workers, lovers, husband, or wife?

Once you've established your greatest values, you can start to shift your time to fit accordingly. You may shine some light on a value you didn't know you had. Or, you might see how much time you've been giving to an activity you don't really value at all. The simple act of awareness is a powerful one. It, in and of itself, can begin to create change. Don't rush the process! Take one thing at a time.

There's a saying that I heard from one of my business partners. Apparently it's popular in the military (he's a former marine and I heard the same saying later from a naval helicopter pilot). It goes like this: "Slow is smooth and smooth is fast." What it means is that if you slow down, you're less likely to make mistakes. If you make a lot of mistakes, you have to go back and fix them, and that takes time; so the best way to save time is actually to slow down. We rush through our lives trying to avoid our own deaths. The irony is funny when think about it. Slow down and pay attention to what you're doing. You're sure to make fewer mistakes, and you might realize you'd be better served doing something else completely.

Another saying I've heard is this: "If you want to understand what a person loves, pay attention to what they give the most time to." The problem I've found with this one is it seems to only really hold up in a world where money isn't an issue. I have worked with plenty of clients who hate what they do for a living, but spend more time working than doing anything else. This brings us to the second major resource category—money.

Money

Money, like time, seems to be one of those things we never have enough of. It is one of the major life-stressors of today and a leading reason for the breakup of many relationships. A healthy relationship with money is essential to your health. They keys to mastering this resource are the same as mastering your health: awareness, education, and discipline.

While we all want more money, we don't all ask ourselves the question of how much more. When is it enough? Here are some questions to ask yourself to help you build more mindfulness around your relationship with money:

- How much money do I want to earn each year?
- How much money do I want to save each year?
- Would I prefer to live with nicer amenities and save less or save more and live with less?
- What do I want to spend my money on?
- What happens when I don't think I have enough money?
- What would happen if I didn't make the money I wanted?
- What amount of time am I willing to give to achieving my financial goals?

I know first hand the trials and troubles money worries can bring. Being an entrepreneur and small-business owner didn't exactly have me rolling in the dough. The loss of security that comes from starting your own business can be quite scary. Especially when you have a family, like I do, that you want to support and take care of. One thing I've come to understand, with much help from my wife, is that you need to be realistic about your relationship with money and its effects on you. This realization helps to instill faith that you're going to be okay. The saints and sages throughout time have warned of the dangers of becoming too attached to material possessions. These are the things money can buy, the creature comforts the world has to offer. In our society, we've decided that the meat and potatoes of life are in financial success, while the gravy is our relationships and spiritual pursuits. It may be wiser to reverse this model and slowly release some of our servitude to money.

"This is all great in theory," you might say, but how do I make it happen? The questions above are a good start; they provide the awareness. Next comes education. If you're not in the field of financial planning, it may be a good idea to higher someone who is, someone who can educate you on your options for retirement savings, short- and long-term investing, life insurance policies, etc. Regardless of whether you hire a professional or not, I recommend creating a personal budget. There is a great software available online called You Need a Budget (www.youneedabudget.com). You can download it to your desktop for free and track all of your monthly expenses and savings goals. The full version with all features only costs $60. You'll save more than that once you start budgeting. The final step is the discipline. This is the hardest part of the model. Once your budget is set, you have your guidelines for spending. It's up to you to stick to them. It might help to set your sights on a vacation you've been meaning to take or maybe a new car or home. Each month you stick to your budget and know that it's getting you closer to this purchase with what you save.

If you're going to function within a society, you need to have a certain degree of mastery over how you spend your time and money. There are always places to be and deadlines to meet. There are always bills to pay and things to do. Until you learn to understand your values and shift your actions to support them, there will also be suffering. Gaining control over time and money not only sets you up for more material success, but also frees you from the mental/emotional anguish these two resources can cause.

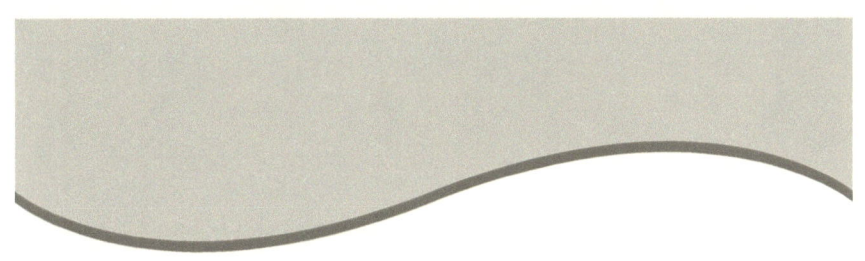

CHAPTER 7

STRESS: EVERYTHING IS STRESSFUL, AND THAT'S A GOOD THING

"Impossible is just a big word thrown around by small men who find it easier to live in the world they've been given than to explore the power they have to change it. Impossible is not a fact. It's an opinion. Impossible is not a declaration it's a dare. Impossible is potential. Impossible is temporary. Impossible is nothing."
– Muhammad Ali

Awareness Questions

1. Are you currently aware of the biggest stressor in your life right now?
2. Do you know what you want to change?
3. Do you know the underlying causes?
4. Do you know what is stopping you from fixing your biggest stressor?
5. Do you understand how your body's physiologic response to stress affects your health?
6. Do you have a system for eliminating or at least minimizing major stressors?
7. Is stress good for you?
8. Are you creating what you truly want in your life?
9. Do you have confidence in yourself and feel that your gifts and talents are good enough to be expressed?
10. Are you comfortable to be yourself fully and openly in a particular relationship, with a specific person?

Education

The seventh key is arguably the most important. All the other elements, in fact all things around us, are influenced by and exist as varying levels of stress. The term when used in the same sentence as health more times than not refers to as a "bad" thing when in fact it is quite important to our overall wellbeing. Stress, when in proper balance, actually makes us stronger. Not only that, but our view of stress, the way we think about it, has a major impact on how it affects our body.

In this chapter I will cover four different categories of stress, how they occur, and what their role is in terms of our health. The last section of the chapter will cover how to balance these categories to ultimately use stress to make you stronger.

Although each category is broken out independently, they are all intimately connected. Think of it like a series of four sinks that are all plumbed together. If one sink is filled to the brim, it will fill the other three sinks until they all level out. Stress in the body can act in a similar way. For example, if your mental/emotional stress is high, then your physical body will be influenced.

Parasympathetic vs. Sympathetic Responses

Before we begin to explore stress and its different categories, I want to explain the system that is responsible for the physiological actions that happen to your body in response to stress. The body's nervous system can be divided into two segments: the somatic or peripheral nervous system, and the autonomic or central nervous system. Arguably there is a third, the enteric nervous system, which relates to digestion, but for the context of this chapter, we will stick with the most common two. The central nervous system can then be further divided into its sympathetic and parasympathetic parts.

The peripheral nervous system is composed of a series of nerves radiating out from the spinal chord to the skeletal muscles, ligaments, and tendons. It is largely responsible for conscious movement, (walking, throwing a ball, even taking a conscious deep breath). The central nervous system is a series of nerves radiating from the spinal column to different organ and glands in the body. Its functioning is done, for the most part, without our conscious control (regulating body temperature, monitoring heart rate, regulating hormones, etc.). The autonomic or central nervous system carries out its functions based on activation or suppression of either the parasympathetic or sympathetic system.

The sympathetic nervous system is sometimes referred to as the fight or flight system. In times of high stress, this system is dominant. A series of physiological responses begin to take place to help prepare the body for a fight or to run from danger. Evolutionarily, this has been a very important system for survival. During times of high stress, the hypothalamus and pituitary gland signal the adrenals to produce a series of hormones, including epinephrine (adrenalin) and cortisol (a stress hormone). These hormones, along with others, increase heart rate and respiration, dilate the pupils, shunt blood from the core to the limbs, and hinder or shut down the digestive and reproductive systems. In situations of short-term stresses, these physiological effects have proven to be essential for survival. However, they are not meant to serve as a sustained solution. If chronic, their effects on our health are devastating. Symptoms can be sporadic, unrelated, and can include depression, insomnia, short temper, energy loss, impaired digestion assimilation and elimination, decreased sex drive, impaired immune function, and irritable bowel syndrome.

Parasympathetic dominance is sometimes referred to as the rest digest system. It works on the opposite cycle of the sympathetic. Interestingly, using a technique like breathing to create a more parasympathetic condition for the respiratory and cardiovascular system has a waterfall effect on the other systems in the body. Meaning, if you're consciously experiencing a sympathetic dominant state, simply pausing and taking a few slow, deep breaths can shift the entire body to a more parasympathetic dominant state. While a parasympathetic dominance may sound more desirable of the two, if out of balance, it too can cause health issues similar to those of a sympathetic dominant state. The ideal is balance. The sympathetic system should be activated from time to time, just like it is with many forms of exercise or mental problem solving, but these bursts should be relatively short and followed by more prolonged periods of parasympathetic/sympathetic harmony.

Physical

Physical stress occurs every day of your life. As you move throughout your day, you experience the stress of gravity against your body. Without this gravitational stress the muscles, bones ligaments, and tendons would atrophy; the body would begin to breakdown. This is why astronauts working in zero-gravity conditions have special exercise equipment to keep their body fit for life when they return to Earth's gravity. If you've ever broken a bone, you've experienced this weakening first hand. Take, for example, a broken arm. The arm would usually be placed within a cast for four to six weeks. When the cast is removed, there is a clear difference between the limb of the broken arm and the limb of the other. Without the stress of daily use, the muscles of the casted arm began to atrophy and breakdown, causing weakness.

Physical stress can be acute or chronic. An acute stress would be considered something like a broken bone or sprained ankle. An outside force has caused the body physical injury (stress) from which it needs to heal. Chronic physical stress can be skeletal and muscular imbalances, inadequate rest, or over training. Another form of physical stress is diet, but that is covered separately under nutritional stressors.

If the body is imbalanced from the standpoint of the skeletal and muscular system, it will be constantly allocating energy to attempt to correct these imbalances. Working with a trained professional to help correct these imbalances can change your life. Recommendations for remedying these conditions are discussed in Chapter Four.

Proper exercise selection and intensity should always be considered when planning your workouts. Understanding your body's current levels of fitness and how well you've balanced the other key elements of breathing, resting, and eating should help you determine if you are ready for a cross-fit workout or would be better suited taking a yin yoga class. I like to balance my intense workouts with less intense ones. If I do a circuit-style weight training routine on day one, I will find a yoga class for day two or three. I also always close all of the group fitness classes I teach with a Tai Chi-like series to help bring the body back to balance after a more intense workout.

Mental/Emotional

In today's society, mental stress is probably one of our greatest sources of chronic stress. Stresses of the past used to be primarily physical, fighting for our survival in a harsh and demanding world. We have now in many ways conquered the demands of the environment. We find ourselves removed almost entirely from it. We have running water in our homes, shelters to cover us from harsh weather conditions, and grocery stores with shelves stocked with food to feed us. The modernized world has eliminated many of the stressors of the past, but there are new enemies in its place. The yoga philosophy outlines six emotional disturbances, which are lust, anger, pride, greed, hatred, and obsession. Their opposites are then sexual restraint, happiness, humility, giving, love, and non-attachment. Practicing these opposites begins to free us from the chains of the mind. One of the things I love about yoga philosophy is the principle that we must learn to become a master of our senses, not a slave to them. We do this by cultivating awareness to our current state and then slowly changing it to a more desirable one. There is no question that this process takes considerable time and thus quite a bit of dedication. The good news is that the changes can be felt almost immediately.

The first step towards eliminating major mental stressors is to take time for reflection. The Buddhist practice of Shamata meditation is great for this. Find a comfortable seat. It can be on a bolster on the ground or in a chair. Close your eyes and take a few deep breaths to center yourself and relax. Keep the body still and begin to pay attention to your breath. Follow the breath from the tip of the nose all the way to the bottom of the pelvic floor and then back out. As thoughts come into your mind, simply recognize them as being there and then let them go. Draw your focus back to your breath. See if you can sit for a few minutes to start and then slowly build up. Eventually Shamata leads to Vipasana, a meditation in which more understanding of the thoughts are reached, but it is best to seek the council of a teacher at that point.

Discipline

Another important step is identifying your major energy drainers (i.e., stressors).

Here's an exercise to help walk you through it. Start with a blank piece of paper and list all of the things currently in your life that drain energy from you. Focus on who or what makes you feel tired, drained, or worn out. Think expansively—it may be a food, scent, building, person, memory, or activity. Once you've got your list, circle your top three. From your top three, underline the number one biggest drainer in your life currently. Then using the model below, begin to develop your plan for either balancing or removing this energy drainer from your life.

Stressor	Causes
• What's not working? • What do you want to change?	• What are the underlying causes? • What's stopping you from fixing it? • Who or what is benefiting from not fixing it?

Outcomes	Effects
• What do you want instead of the problem / stress?	• What will it do for you to eliminate this stress? • What will you learn from it? • How will reaching the desired outcome change things?

Resources
• What skills, capabilities, states, information, equipment, contacts etc. do you have that will help you to solve the current stress? • Have you faced a problem like this before? If so how did you solve it?

The SCORE method is really an exercise in critical thinking, but can be quite effective in helping to understand a current stressor and its effects and then to navigate solutions to put the stressor back into balance. Using the questions listed in each box of the diagram to the left, walk yourself through the current stressor. Be as specific as possible. If applicable, include dates and times.

Nutritional

Nutrition has been covered in great detail in the beginning chapters of this book. The effects of nutrition are largely chemical and absolutely contribute in some way to all other systems. Eating appropriately for your biochemical individuality and becoming more attuned to your body's needs are crucial to total health. Other than being aware of the physical effects nutrition can have, we can also cultivate some mindfulness around the way we eat. In this section I will offer a list of activities worth trying at mealtime to help cultivate a more holistic approach to eating. They are as follows.

- Eat in a settled atmosphere. Avoid TV. Sit down to eat.
- Never eat when you are upset. Stress negatively affects your digestion and can leave you feeling worse than before you ate.
- Eat when you feel hungry. Know the difference between hunger and cravings. Often, people mistake hunger for lack of hydration. Try drinking a glass of good clean water first.
- Avoid ice-cold food and drink. Your body has to work harder to warm food/drink to a proper temperature for healthy digestion.
- Eat at a moderate pace, neither too fast nor too slow. Chew your food to an almost liquid consistency. This will make your food more easily digestible and optimize nutrient intake.

- Wait until one meal is digested before eating the next.
- Eat freshly cooked meals whenever possible. Reduce FLNC (frozen, leftover, nuked, canned).
- Experience all six tastes at every meal: sour, sweet, salty, pungent, bitter, and astringent. Leave one-quarter of your stomach empty to aid digestion.
- Sit quietly for a few minutes after your meal. Take a walk if you can.
- Add a pinch of Celtic sea salt to your water.

Chemical

Chemical stressors are found in the foods we eat, the drinks we consume, and the environment in which we move. We live in a world that is full of chemical additives, preservatives, colorings, fresheners, softeners, cleaners, and beautifiers. Many of these chemicals are toxic to the human body and can lead to serious health issues. The thing is, oftentimes we encounter these chemicals in such small doses that it takes repeated exposure to them over long periods of time to really "feel" anything. When you do finally feel something, symptoms can seem unrelated or can be misdiagnosed. Because of this delay in effect, chemical stressors are often written off or never even taken into consideration as a threat to your health. For a list of common household sources of chemical stressors, refer back to Chapter Five. For a list of common nutritional chemical stressors, refer to Chapter One. Removing additional chemical stress is important for effective functioning of your cells. The less toxic material the body is forced to clean out, the more the body can use that energy for higher-order needs.

CONCLUSION: THE MEANING OF LIFE

It has become the stereotypical philosophical question: what is the meaning of life? While a good question, I think it isn't the question most people really want the answer to. The meaning of life is universal. In other words, it is the same for everyone. Ready? Here it is. The meaning of life is to perform the actions of your life for the betterment of humanity. That's it. Imagine if everyone on planet earth did that! What would this world look like?

The more difficult question to answer, and the one I think most people would rather have the answer to, is this: what is my purpose in life, or stated a bit differently, how do I fulfill life's meaning? This is not so universal. There are many ways in which you can contribute to the betterment of humanity. There are many ways in which you can't as well. Wisdom is knowing the difference and having the discipline to act accordingly. This is the question people want answered when they ask for life's meaning. They're really asking, "What is my purpose?" or "How do I fulfill the innate desire to help improve the world I'm a part of?"

Me? I'm very fortunate. I believe the meaning of life is what I stated it to be above, but more importantly, I know my purpose. I hope this book serves as a piece of that purpose, a written word that in some way helps the person who picks it up and reads it.

I've spent years reading, practicing, and testing what it means to live a healthy life. This book is a summary of a lot of that work, a pretty concise road map that highlights what I feel to be the seven key topics worth addressing and how to address them. Follow the AED model: awareness, education, and discipline. Tune in, learn, and adjust the quantity and quality of these key elements while balancing your environment, maximizing your resources, and concurring your stressors. If you can do this, you've built the foundation needed to fulfill your purpose. Health builds vitality. Vitality is the wellspring of energy. Energy is needed for anything and everything you do. Without the energy to complete a task, your purpose remains a distant concept set up for its future seat in your mind as the "thing you wished you'd done." Don't let your purpose slip by. Maximize your health, build vitality and energy, and go change the world!

ABOUT THE AUTHOR

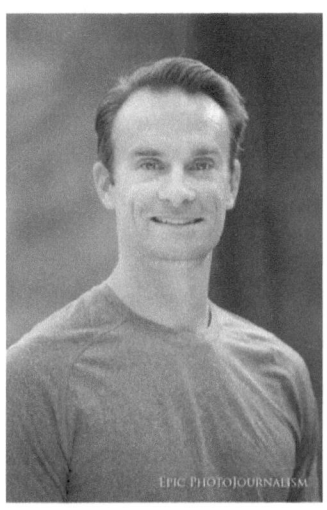

For nearly a decade, Ryan's passion has been to identify and learn the best services, methods, and philosophies that support and nurture the health and wellness of human beings. He and his partners started MOSAIC as a way to share this knowledge in an attempt to empower leaders who embody health, wisdom, and soul.

Ryan has studied at the National Academy of Sports Medicine, the CHEK Institute for advanced performance, the Metabolic Typing Education Center, and Symmetry's school for alignment therapy. He recognizes health as the balance and synergy of the human body's many systems.

Additionally, Ryan is a 200-hour Yoga Alliance registered yoga teacher. For him, yoga is the way of the warrior. The warrior spirit is conscious of its thoughts and actions. Its focus is sharp and clear, and it displays tolerance and understanding for all things, especially itself. When Ryan steps onto his mat to guide a class, he brings with him his warrior spirit.

Ryan is the team lead for MOSAIC Health. He also leads MOSAIC's yoga teacher training, health workshops, and co-facilitates some of MOSAIC's leadership programs. He works one-on-one with private clients and is the creator of MOSAIC's Good Being, Good Living Holistic Health program.

MOSAIC Institute for Human Development LLC
811 25th St. Suite 102
San Diego CA. 92102
info@exploremosaic.com
www.exploremosaic.com

REFERENCES

1   Iyengar, B.K.S. *Light On Pranayama*. New York: The Crossroad Publishing Company, 2012.

2   Wikipedia Contributors. "Old MacDonald Had a Farm." *Wikipedia, The Free Encyclopedia*. http://en.wikipedia.org/w/index.php?title=Special: Cite&page=Old_MacDonald_Had_a_Farm&id=626844782. (accessed 6 October 2014).

3   Lucett, Scott C., ed. *NASM Essentials of Personal Fitness Training*, 3rd ed. Baltimore: Lippincott Williams & Wilkins, 2007.

4   Center for Diesease Controll and Prevention, *Adult Obesity Facts*, 28th March 2014, 24th June 2014 <http://www.cdc.gov/obesity/data/adult.html>.

5   Mortimer J. Adler. *A Guidebook to Learning*. New York: Macmillan Publishing Company, 1986.

6   Mortimer J. Adler. *A Guidebook To Learning*. New York: Macmillan Publishing Company, 1986.

7   Walsh, Bryan P. "The Gut Fat Loss Connection," Rescue My Health LLC. http://fatisnotyourfault.com/blog2/wp-content/uploads/2011/11/finyf_gut_supplement.pdf.

8   Chek, Paul. *How to Eat, Move and Be Healthy!* San Diego: CHEK Institute, 2004.

9   Erasmus, Udo. *Fats that Heal Fats that Kill*. Summertown, TN: Alive Books, 1993. 4.

10 Balch, Phyllis A. *Prescriptions for Nutritional Healing: The A-to-Z Guide to Supplements*. New York: Avery Trade, 2008.

11 Freudenrich, Craig. "How Fat Cells Work." 27 October 2000. HowStuffWorks. com. http://health.howstuffworks.com/human-body/cells-tissues/fat-cell.htm.

12 HowStuffWorks.com. "Is There a Way to Compare a Human Being to an Engine in Terms of Efficiency." 05 December 2000. http://auto.howstuffworks.com/question527.htm.

13 Nienhiser, Jill. "Characteristics of Traditional Diets." *The Weston A Price Foundation*. 1 January 2000. http://www.westonaprice.org/health-topics/abcs-of-nutrition/characteristics-of-traditional-diets/.

14 "Fallon, Sally M., and Thomas S. Cowan, MD. The Nourishing Traditions Book of Baby & Child Care

15 Chek, Paul. *How to Eat, Move and Be Healthy!* San Diego: CHEK Institute, 2004.

16 Wolcott, William. *The Metabolic Typing Diet.* New York: Broadway Books, 2000.

17 Pollan, Michael. *Cooked.* New York: Penguin Books, 2014.

18 Pollan, Michael. "How Cooking Can Change Your Life." YouTube, 4 September 2013. https://www.youtube.com/watch?v=TX7kwfE3cJQ.

19 Kirschmann, John D. and Inc. Nutriiton Search. *Nutrition Almanac.* New York: McGraw-Hill Books, 2007.

20 Lipski, Elizabeth. *Digestive Wellness*, Vol. 3 .New York: McGraw-Hill, 2005.

21 Coulter, H. David. *Anatomy of Hatha Yoga: A Manual for Students, Teachers and Practitioners.* Albany: Body & Breath, 2001.

22 Coulter, H. David. *The Anatomy of Hatha Yoga.* Albany: Body & Breath Inc., 2001.

23 Keach, Stephanie. *The Yoga Handbook.* Ashville: Stephanie and Sunny Keach, 2003.

24 Robin, Mel. *A Handbook for Yogasana Teachers: The incorporation of Neuroscience, Physiology, and Anatomy into the Practice.* Tucson: Wheatmark, 2009.

25 Wolcott, William, and Trish Fahey. *The Metabolic Typing Diet.* New York: Broadway Books, 2000.

26 National Sleep Foundation. *Sleep-Wake Cycle: Its Physiology and Impact on Health*, National Sleep Foundation. Washington DC: National Sleep Foundation, 2006.

27 National Sleep Foundation, *Sleep-Wake Cycle: Its Physiology and Impact on Health*, National Sleep Foundation (DC: Nationla Sleep Foundation, 2006).

28 Wiley, T.S. and Bent Formby, *Lights Out: Sleep, Sugar, and Survival.* New York: Pocket Books, 2000.

29 Robin, Mel. *A Handbook for Yogasana Teachers: The Incorporation of Neuroscience, Physiology, and Anatomy into the Practice.* Tucson: Wheatmark, 2009.

30 Robin, Mel. *A Handbook for Yogasana Teachers: The Incorporation of Neuroscience, Physiology, and Anatomy into the Practice.* Tucson: Wheatmark, 2009.

31 Mummy, Patrick. *Symmetry Complete Level 3: A Practitioners Guide to Postural Alignment Therapy.* Folsom, CA: Symmetry for Healthn.d.

32 Mummy, Patrick. *Symmetry Complete Level 3: A Practitioners Guide to Postural Alignment Therapy.* Folsom, CA: Symmetry for Healthn.d.

33 Lucett, Scott C., ed. *NASM Essentials of Personal Fitness Training,* 3rd ed. Baltimore: Lippincott Williams & Wilkins, 2007.

34 Long, Ray. *The Key Poses of Yoga.* Champlain, NY: Bandha Yoga Publications LLC, 2008.

35 Chek, Paul. *Movement that Matters.* Vista, CA: Paul Chek, 2011.

36 Hartley, Linda. *Wisdom of the Body Moving: An Introduction to Body-Mind Centering.* Berkeley: North Atlantic Books, 1995.

37 Hartley, Linda. *Wisdom of the Body Moving: An Introduction to Body-Mind Centering.* Berkeley: North Atlantic Books, 1995.

38 Chek, Paul. *Primal Pattern Movements.* Vista, CA: CHEK Institute, 2011.

INDEX